Peter Stemmet is an award-winning broadcaster and blogger. He is a sports presenter at Al Jazeera in Doha, Qatar. Previously he worked in television news, including eNCA, in his native South Africa. Stemmet's work over the years has included presenting, reporting, scripting, sub-editing, producing, and interviewing the world's top sports personalities. In addition to television, Stemmet is also a master of ceremonies, voice artist, freelance writer/blogger, and part-time broadcasting lecturer. He received in June 2009 the SAB Sports News Reporter of the Year Award. In 2015 he landed the SA Blog Awards Sports Blog of the Year accolade.

Dedicated to my wonderful wife, Ntando, and beautiful daughters, Hannah and Eden.

Peter Stemmet

How to Become a Sports Journalist

AUSTIN MACAULEY PUBLISHERS®

LONDON * CAMBRIDGE * NEW YORK * SHARJAH

A CIP catalogue record for this title is available from the British Library.

ISBN 9781035809363 (Paperback)
ISBN 9781035809370 (ePub e-book)

www.austinmacauley.com

First Published 2024
Austin Macauley Publishers Ltd®
1 Canada Square
Canary Wharf
London
E14 5AA

Firstly, thanks and praise be to God Almighty, the Creator of the Universe. Thank you for blessing me with this talent to be able to do a job that brings me joy. I know I can never love You as much as You love me, but I will not stop trying.

Thank you to my wife Ntando for your enduring support and encouragement. Ngiyakuthanda!

To my daughters Hannah and Eden, the sports nut inside of me hopes you grow up to become a WTA or LPGA superstar but if your interests and talents lie elsewhere that will also be okay. Daddy loves you both very much!

To my parents Piet and Delene, thank you for always believing in me and willing me on to be the best that I can be. I love you both endlessly.

To my uncle Klaus, no one has been as responsible for nurturing my love of sport as you, thank you (even if you did cheat in our backyard cricket matches. What kind of an adult man bullies a 10-year-old kid in a game of garden cricket, anyway?) I love you in spite of this.

To my sister Melissa, who spent many hours in the backyard playing sports with me too (sometimes on Klaus' side. Imagine ganging up on a preteen like that!) I love you always.

To my other family members Baba Bheki, Mum Tshengi, Lungelo Chonco, Zama Chonco, Caron Münch, Charien O'Connor, Ouma Stemmet, my uncle and aunties Stemmet: Emmerentia, Hennie, Marlene, Petro, Mauritz, Coreen and all my cousins, especially Aiden for helping with the book cover selection and my wonderful godchild Emily. All my love.

I also want to thank some of my old university lecturers. Stijn Postema, Rachel Dungar and Simon Pia: Thank you for believing in me and always being full of encouragement. To the late Alan Simmonds, it upsets me that I only met you so late in your life, but I am so glad I did. Thank you for everything. Lots of love from me to you.

To Roi Simpson and Neil Ovens. I know I have said this at least 999 times (and I'll say it another 99 000) but without your help and guidance all those years ago who knows where I would have ended up? Thank you for helping me start my career in broadcasting. Love you guys!

I also want to mention my friends who have always stood by me and one way or another assisted with this book too. They are Bertus Hugo, Jean-Pierre Lopion, Kanyiso Colani, Mike Franck, Patrick Franck, Martin Myers, Andrew D'Ercole, Michael Marillier, David Ward, Jannie Stemmet (not related but he is a Stemmet so obviously a cool guy), Eric Roest, Mark Lee, Francois Brill and Jaco Brill. Believe it or not, I love you all!

Finally, I also have to thank my beloved pet, toy Pomeranian Zulu, for lying at my feet for many of the hours I spent writing this book. I love you, boy.

I have no doubt I have forgotten somebody and no doubt will remember your name after this book is published. I can only beg for your mercy and forgiveness.

Table of Contents

Chapter One
Kicking Off

I love sport. As a young boy, I watched all the matches that were on the television and this trend continued as I became a teenager, a young adult and now a married man with a young daughter. I used to wake up early in the morning, or stay up late at night, to watch games.

In 1994, at the age of 11, my mum allowed me to stay up to watch the football World Cup final between Brazil and Italy. It was being played in California and factoring in the time difference, kick off was only at about 21:30 in South Africa and I had to go to school the next day.

I was grateful and thought I had a "cool Mum". Her "coolness" was stretched to its very limits when the match went into extra time and a penalty shootout! I think I only went to sleep well after midnight. I would have been devastated if my old lady had forced me to go to bed at my regular time that night.

My love of sport did not just consist of watching games on the TV. I joined my school's various sports teams and even signed up at a local club when my school did not offer a certain sport, like football for example. Unfortunately for me, my dreams were quickly dashed when it became painfully apparent that I lacked any real talent.

My on-field exploits might well make for an embarrassing, cringe worthy comedy. However, I did have a handful of happy memories, even if they were as rare as vibranium from the Black Panther comics.

My primary school thought of me as such an impressive youngster that they made me their vice-head boy. This leadership position paid off when I was made captain of the Under-13 cricket "B" team I played for. In my first match as skipper, I won the toss and decided to bat first.

My naïve logic suggested the cracks in the pitch would widen and make batting more difficult for our opponents. That would almost certainly have been the logic of South Africa's cricket captain at the time, Hansie Cronje, so who could blame me for attempting to emulate him?

However, no one told me that that pitch had been played on for years without any meaningful maintenance. Furthermore, I was blissfully unaware that pre-teens were unlikely to take advantage of any cracks in the surface anyway, let alone bowl with the venom necessary to cause even further damage to the playing surface.

We put up a half-decent score, but I knew we would have to bowl well if we were going to defend it. I gathered the boys in a huddle and tried my best to deliver a motivational speech that would rally the troops. Despite us taking wickets at regular intervals, I could sense the match was slowly slipping away from us.

As the team's leader, I took the decision to bring myself on to bowl. Even though hitherto, none of my coaches, or captains, had shown any faith in my bowling ability, I knew I could bowl. I had been bowling in backyards across Cape Town for years, not to mention the nets during practice sessions with relative success.

I walked up to my mark and began jogging in to deliver my first ever gentle medium pacer. The ball pitched outside the batsman's off stump and moved a little bit away from him as he attempted a cover drive. For the purposes of this anecdote, we shall say that it was a beautiful away swinger that Vernon Philander would have been proud of.

Sure enough, the batsman made contact with the ball, but only in the form of an outside edge-just like a typical "Big Vern" victim. My friend Bradley Bell, who I had been playing backyard cricket with for years, was fielding at first slip. As the captain, I had placed him there because I knew he was a very capable fielder.

The ball headed towards Bradley who positioned his hands beautifully in front of his face and clutched the ball. It was safe and secure in his palms and I jubilantly hared over to him to give him the biggest hug ever. I had taken a wicket with the first ball I had ever bowled in a cricket match.

I would never go on to achieve anything else in sport, but that remains a treasured memory. Thank you, Bradley, for not dropping that ball!

I tried out as a goalkeeper in football, but I accepted the writing was probably on the wall after we lost a preseason friendly 11-0! Even so, we played one game where I pulled off some really spectacular saves, and just for that one day, I felt like a hero. Sadly, there was not much else to celebrate in my football career, or any other sport I attempted to play for that matter.

Over the years, I also tried playing tennis, rugby, golf, squash, baseball, track and field athletics, field hockey and basketball. I am nothing more than average male height so Heaven only knows what I thought I might achieve on the basketball court.

I can only imagine men like Michael Jordan and LeBron James licking their lips at the prospect of finding themselves one-on-one with me in the paint.

Perhaps you can relate to this. Maybe you also tried playing a variety of sports in the hope of making a career out of it; amateur or professional, but you just did not have the requisite talent. Possibly you were slightly better than that and made your way into a decent local club team, but you were never quite good enough to play at the next level.

After accepting that being a sportsman or woman was not going to be your destiny, you decided that maybe another way to work in sport was to become a sports journalist. If this sounds remotely relatable, then keep reading. This book has been written for you.

This is the very category that I fall into myself. It is important to note that this book is not a substitute for a university degree. Instead, it should be regarded as a supplementary guide with practical tips on how to take what you have already learnt and better put it into practice.

I have met many young people during my career who came straight out of university and after seeing them in action for just a few minutes, wondered to myself what they had been taught in the last three or so years. In some cases, I had even quietly thought to myself that perhaps this youngster should go back to the tertiary education institution and ask for their money back.

The aim of this book is to help you and equip you with practically useful information that for whatever reason they are not giving you at university.

As I write this, I have worked across radio, television, magazines, newspapers and digital media in the area of sports reporting and presenting over a period of 19 years. I am going to share my personal story with you in this book as well as advice on how you can go on to have a successful career and be the very best in your field.

Your journey is unlikely to be exactly like mine but by sharing my story, I hope you will get a good understanding of how to go about things and get a sense of what is possible.

Along the way, you are also going to read the thoughts and advice of several respected sports journalists who have decades of experience across the various platforms. In this book, you will hear from *Outkick* senior NFL writer Armando Salguero, television producers Brian Gleeson and Raymond Herbst, former *Sky Sports New Zealand* Head of Sport Craig Norenbergs, broadcast sports journalist and founder of *African Sports Content Network* Junia Stainbank, sports photographer Lefty Shivambu, worldwide IRONMAN announcer Paul Kaye, sports news freelancer Paul Rhys, football commentator Peter Drury, *ESPN Cricinfo* editor-in-chief Sambit Bal and *Hashtag Our Stories (*now known as *Seen)* co-founder Yusuf Omar, as well as sports lawyers, Andrew Nixon, Exavier Pope and Larry Fenelon.

Let me also warn you that sports journalism is no longer just about being a reporter who attends a match on a Saturday, writes a wrap report and then attends the team's next pre-match press conference later in the week. Assignments are considerably more detailed than that and with shrinking budgets now almost universal, the demand for multi-skilled journalists with a wealth of general knowledge is only increasing.

This is what you are going to want to become and I, along with this book's guests, will share with you how to become that journalist.

In 2004, when I started at a community radio station in the town of Paarl, north of Cape Town in South Africa, it was not actually as a sports journalist. I was the host of a music entertainment show on a Saturday morning. That was my real dream in fact; to become a radio presenter.

I graduated from Saturday mornings to afternoon drive prime time after about five months. I knew an afternoon drive show needed more elements than just good music, entertainment news and some colourful stories. News, sport, weather and traffic updates were incorporated and since I was a big sports fan anyway, I largely took care of the sports element in the show myself.

On Wednesdays and Fridays, I was joined by a local mechanic, Henry (who also loved sport), for a full hour of sports coverage. Henry was a Paarlite and had access to the local sports teams as well as good relationships with many of the players and coaches.

Since I was not actually from Paarl and driving in every day from Cape Town, our agreement was that he would take care of local sport and I would be in charge of the stuff that was of a more national and international nature. It worked very well, and we had many local club players and coaches on our show.

Henry arranged all of these while I was more of an observer, not quite fully grasping how I was partaking in journalism without consciously being a journalist.

After 15 months at Radio KC, I joined P4 Radio as a sports anchor on their afternoon drive. They had a vacancy that I applied for and after a successful rehearsal, I was given the job on the spot. My initial intention was to take this job as my way in and eventually move on to being a proper music entertainment presenter.

After four months, I began hosting shows on P4 when other presenters were unavailable. Over a three-year period, in which P4 changed its name to Heart 104.9, I was the sports anchor on the afternoon drive show, and the station's go-to stand-in host. Eventually, I was given the Weekend Breakfast show.

I had a sports hour on a Saturday morning with a man named Martin Myers, who subsequently became a dear friend. It was not really journalism, but more a case of banter, although Martin did regularly bring in guests. So, similar to my scenario with Henry, I was participating in sports journalism without actually consciously being a journalist.

I was also moved from the afternoon drive to a specific slot for a 30-minute daily sports feature, called The Sports Cage. This was not particularly challenging as it was externally produced and the interview audio clips were emailed to us ahead of time. All I really did was present the show and introduce two feature interviews.

I did not really mind at all because I was still more focused on being an out-and-out radio presenter but then in May 2008, my world came crashing down. I was called in by the programme manager and told I was being taken off the Weekend Breakfast show.

My dreams were shattered. I became depressed, despondent and desperate. After phoning every commercial radio station in South Africa in the hope of landing alternative employment, and even having a meeting with the programme manager at Kfm, Heart's rival radio station, I was unable to find what I was looking for.

As it turned out, I happened to share my story with a former colleague of mine, Robin Adams. Robin and I met about a year earlier when he was the Breakfast Show producer at Heart 104.9 in the week, and a sports journalist on weekends at eTV. He regularly encouraged me to join him in television, but I was adamant that I was a radio guy.

As it turned out, eTV had just launched a 24-hour news channel, e News Channel, and they had a vacancy for a sports reporter. By then, things had changed sufficiently in my own personal circumstances and when he mentioned this vacancy to me, I did not hesitate to apply.

For the first time in my career, I was going to be an actual sports journalist. There was a lot I did not know or understand. I had never worked in television, for example, and I was certainly not used to attending press conferences, but I was determined to learn as quickly as I could, and I immersed myself in my new role.

In a five-year period at e News Channel, I was blessed to cover a football World Cup, Africa Cup of Nations, Tri-Nations rugby, Champions Trophy and Indian Premier League cricket, Afro Basket qualifiers, Davis Cup and SA Open tennis, Dakar Rally testing and an Olympic Games. That is not a bad list by any standard and if it seems exciting to you, let me tell you it is merely the tip of the iceberg.

In 2012, e News Channel rebranded and became eNCA. Funny how the places I work at change their names! Eventually, I left eNCA and joined a start-up channel, ANN7. The channel itself had a disastrous launch and owing to political interference and biases, lacked any real credibility.

It was difficult working there but equally challenging was having to explain why I was working there when people found out I was employed at the channel.

What working at ANN7 did give me was more in-studio screen time. At eNCA, I was a reporter who occasionally anchored bulletins; usually when people were sick or on leave. But at ANN7, I was the prime time sports anchor.

I worked there for three years and in that time, I also hosted sports magazine shows around the football, rugby and cricket world cups, and I even branched out into current affairs and became a regular host of the prime time news bulletin, while also hosting a U.S. elections weekly magazine show.

That was the U.S. election won ultimately by Donald Trump, so it was a very colourful experience as you can imagine.

No doubt ANN7, for all its faults, was a move that worked out well for me in terms of building up regular screen time and it was truly a case of going one step backward in order to take two steps forward when I left the troubled television news channel to join the world-renowned news network, Al Jazeera as a sports presenter.

I went from working at a place that struggled for credibility to a channel with a global reputation for excellence. Interestingly, ANN7 would go on to change their name, so yet another name change, although I had already left by then.

Outside of my radio and television work, I had also written articles for several magazines and newspapers, as well as online publications, although in each case, it was only as a freelancer. In this book, I shall share with you how to work as a sports journalist in a freelance capacity as well as in the newer fields that have emerged in the last few years like podcasting and YouTube shows.

In 2016, I hosted my own podcast but it only lasted 10 episodes. Why did it stop? Well, episode 10 happened to coincide with my joining Al Jazeera, so I dropped it there and then. The podcast itself was part of a larger media house I started called The Sports Eagle. It was a sports news website and in this book, I shall also share lessons from the digital journalism sphere.

If all of this sounds like just the kind of thing that you want to be part of and you need to know more, then turn the page and let's get this journey started and allow me to help you become the very best sports journalist you can be.

Chapter Two
Sport Is a Big Deal, It Needs Journalism

Before we sink our teeth into why sport needs journalism, let us define the art first. Dictionary.com says journalism is, "the occupation of reporting, writing, editing, photographing, or broadcasting news or of conducting any news organisation as a business".

That is going to help us at a later stage when we delve into the different types of journalists that exists. The online dictionary further defines journalism as, "writing that reflects superficial thought and research, a popular slant, and hurried composition, conceived of as exemplifying topical newspaper or popular magazine writing as distinguished from scholarly writing".[1]

Moreover, journalism is the activity of gathering, assessing, creating, and presenting news and information. It is also the product of these activities. It can be distinguished from other activities and products by certain identifiable characteristics and practices.

These elements not only separate journalism from other forms of communication, they are what make it indispensable to democratic societies. History reveals that the more democratic a society, the more news and information it tends to have. That is according to the American Press Institute.[2]

Every journalism professor's worst enemy, and at the same time every reporter's secret friend, Wikipedia, defines journalism as the production and distribution of reports on current or past events. The word journalism applies to

---

[1] www.dictionary.com. (n.d.). Definition of journalism | Dictionary.com. [online] Available at: https://www.dictionary.com/browse/journalism?s=t.

[2] American Press Institute (2019). What is journalism? Definition and meaning of the craft. [online] American Press Institute. Available at:
https://www.americanpressinstitute.org/journalism-essentials/what-is-journalism/.

the occupation, as well as citizen journalists who gather and publish information. Journalistic media include print, television, radio, Internet, and in the past, newsreels.

Concepts of the appropriate role for journalism vary between countries. In some nations, the news media are controlled by government intervention and are not fully independent. In others, the news media are independent of the government and instead operate as private industry motivated by profit.

In addition to the varying nature of how media organisations are run and funded, countries may have differing implementations of laws handling the freedom of speech and libel cases.[3]

I especially liked the American Press Institute's definition and despite its reputation for unreliability, the Wikipedia definition was not only spot on but thorough too. As you can tell, there are various styles and interpretations to journalism, so ultimately you would have to decide where you fit in.

Since you are reading this, it is safe for me to assume sports journalism is your choice and no doubt, you have already told anyone who will listen that you intend to become a sports journalist. It is unlikely you have the support of everyone who has heard your story, especially your peers intending to become current affairs reporters.

There is a likelihood that they will provide you with mixed feedback. After all, journalism is a profoundly serious profession. Wars, elections, coups d'état, embezzlement, money laundering, racketeering, maladministration and corruption, trumps some football team winning some or other trophy, right?

Not so fast.

The first problem with that kind of thinking is that it assumes, rather naïvely that sport is exclusively about teams or players contesting matches against one another. Nothing could be further from the truth.

Firstly, sport intersects many different industries such as media, construction, real estate, tourism, retail, and even education. This makes it an ideal vehicle to expose mass audiences to new ideas and cross-pollinate emerging technologies into other sectors.

In 2002, Japan and South Korea hosted the FIFA World Cup. It was the first time the event was taking place in Asia and then-president of FIFA, Sepp Blatter

---

[3] Wikipedia Contributors (2019). Journalism. [online] Wikipedia. Available at: https://en.wikipedia.org/wiki/Journalism.

was concerned about interest in the Korean Republic waning if the host nation were to be eliminated.

Half-empty stadiums would not look good on the television, especially when the world's TV networks were paying massive amounts of money for the rights to broadcast the tournament. The Koreans had done very well in the group stages where they finished top of the standings ahead of Poland, Portugal and the United States of America.

However, in the first round of the knockout stage, they would face a considerably more challenging opponent; three-time world champions, Italy. Most experts agreed that it was virtually impossible for the home team to overcome the mighty Italians, who two years prior, finished as runners-up at the European Championships, and would go on to win the World Cup for a fourth time in 2006 in Germany.

Aware of the negative implications a South Korean exit might have on the optical aspect of the tournament, Blatter hatched a plan. The Swiss paid off the match officials, headed by referee Byron Moreno of Ecuador, to ensure that the hosts would progress to the next round.

This only became public knowledge many years later but at the time, South Korea's 2-1 extra time win over the Azzurri was celebrated as one of the World Cup's great all-time upset victories, except in Italy, where the players, coaching staff, federation and fans were justifiably livid.

In the next round, the hosts met Spain, not as decorated an opponent as the Italians, but a formidable foe nevertheless. Thanks to Blatter's generosity, victory was ensured for the home team, courtesy of Egyptian referee, Gamal Ghandour and linesman, Michael Ragoonath of Trinidad and Tobago, the same nation as FIFA vice-president, Jack Warner, who we shall discuss later in this chapter.

Despite the Spaniards scoring two seemingly legal goals, they were both ruled out by the referee and his assistant. Ghandour even blew the full-time whistle one minute ahead of time before the Koreans eliminated Spain in a penalty shootout to reach the semi-finals, where they were defeated by Germany.

No wonder Ghandour's Wikipedia page describes him as "infamous". The Germans won that semi-final match to end South Korea's supposedly dream run, but it will come as no surprise to you that that fixture was the last match of the tournament to be played in South Korea as the final was staged in Japan.[4]

---

[4] Jennings, A. (2016). The dirty game: uncovering the scandal at FIFA. London: Arrow Books. (pp 120-121)

The South Korean players were celebrated for their miraculous exploits. What a magnificent achievement it was for this team, that in its previous history had never even won a match at the World Cup, to go all the way to the semi-finals and what's more, they did it in front of their own supporters on home turf.

If only it was real.

South African football fans have every right to be angry when wondering why Blatter did not extend their country the same courtesy and pay off the match officials in 2010 to ensure that their national team, nicknamed Bafana Bafana, did not become the first host nation in World Cup history to be eliminated in the first round.

After all, he did it for the Koreans, why not for the first African host nation in World Cup history? The difference was that stadiums in South Africa would be quite full whether the home team was playing or not.

Would Bafana Bafana fans have cared if they were to discover 10 years later that their team reaching the knockout stage was an act of crookery? My guess is the reaction would probably initially consist of the modern-day ostensibly obligatory outrage on social media before most people calmed down and turned their attention to more pressing matters.

The truth is that what Blatter did was nothing other than bribery and corruption. If the president of a country was found to have bribed public officials to ensure a favourable outcome for his government administration or to rig an election, it would most certainly be big news. What Blatter did was no different and sadly, sport is full of villains like him and his associates.

While we are on the topic of the 2010 FIFA World Cup that was staged in South Africa, did you know that the FIFA committee responsible for awarding the hosting rights, had actually intended to award that honour to Morocco?

The fact that the South Africans had a superior bid; it was described as "excellent" by the same FIFA inspection group that called the Moroccan bid "very good", did not matter until one Jack Warner of the Confederation of North, Central American and Caribbean Association Football (CONCACAF) proposed a $10 million donation to the FIFA World Cup Diaspora Legacy Programme.

Warner hails from Trinidad and Tobago and while I support democracy, and the free market principle of being able to work your way up the ladder from even the lowest of starting points, it was rather curious that someone from Trinidad and Tobago, hardly what you would describe as a footballing powerhouse, rose the ranks to become a FIFA vice-president.

The Caribbean is home to a large African diaspora population and this donation would go towards developing football for those of African descent who play the sport. What a lovely story. Except that the donation would be made in exchange for Warner and his CONCACAF associates voting for South Africa instead of Morocco, come World Cup hosting rights awarding time.

That donation, while ostensibly well-intended, was nothing but a bribe and it paid dividends. South Africa's bid defeated its Moroccan rival by 14 votes to 10. Had Warner not been adequately greased, and the three CONCACAF votes went Morocco's way, South Africa would have lost out 13-11.[5]

Politicians bribe and are bribed. Sporting administrators do the same. Sporting administrators are politicians. It is important that you start to view them as such. Your favourite team's chairman, president or CEO is not necessarily some benevolent boyhood fan of your club. He or she is a politician. Treat them with the suspicion they merit.

By the way, if you were the South African bid committee, what would you have done? You had the best bid but unless you were willing to make that "donation", you were guaranteed to lose.

As for Warner, well at the time of writing, he was fighting corruption charges in the United States. One of the charges alleged that Warner received a bribe of $5 million to vote for Russia to host the 2018 World Cup.

You might also like to know that despite being awarded the rights to host the 1994 World Cup, the United States of America was in serious danger of missing out on qualifying for the preceding tournament in Italy. As it would turn out, in November 1989, Warner's home nation was up against the U.S. in the final World Cup qualifier for the 1990 tournament.

At the time, the Trinidadians were considered the favourites but FIFA was concerned that the 1990 World Cup needed the presence of the States to help promote the tournament they would be hosting four years later. Having them in Italy would help garner media interest and hopefully, shore up excitement among Americans, who certainly at the time, viewed "soccer" as a much smaller sport.

FIFA could not afford to have the USA absent from the 1990 World Cup. You can probably guess what happened next. A plan was hatched. Warner

---

[5] Hartley, R. (2016). The big fix: how South Africa stole the World Cup. Johannesburg: Jonathan Ball Publishers. (pp 38-67)

arranged for a change in match officials shortly before the game and it paid off handsomely as the U.S. were victorious 1-0.[6]

The yanks were on their way to Italia 90 at the expense of Trinidad and Tobago. Warner conspired against his own country. You might say he had no obligation to be a patriot. Perhaps, but he also conspired against his own national federation and regional federations; federations of which he was a president or vice-president. What a nice guy.

In May 2015, Warner was one of 14 defendants charged in connection with a 24-year scheme to allegedly "enrich themselves through the corruption of international soccer". In September of that year, he was banned from all football activities for life by FIFA.[7]

At least FIFA were being proactive you might say. Maybe but Warner had already quit football more than four years earlier. It was rather more convenient to ban someone who was in effective retirement than actually act against them while they were in your ranks.

It is possible that you might think that men like Blatter and Warner represented the minority and even if these people were criminals, it was probably a lot better in the old days. How often have you heard your parents or grandparents tell you how much better things were in the old days?

Yes, in the old days, sport was run by men of honour. Men like Juan Antonio Samaranch, for example. Samaranch was a cunning character and he did not even invent the tricks of the trade. Instead the Spaniard, who was once a fervent and active Blue Shirt-wearing member of Spain's dictator, General Francisco Franco's fascist *Movimiento* movement, learnt the dark ways of sports administration from Brazil's João Havelange.

The Brazilian, who was head of FIFA, helped Samaranch team up with a German named Horst Dassler, who was the son of Adolf Dassler. If that fact means nothing to you, why not take the first few letters of Adolf and Dassler, and form a new word, like say, Adidas.

---

[6] Jennings, A. (2016). The dirty game: uncovering the scandal at FIFA. London: Arrow Books. (p 113)

[7] Sky Sports. (n.d.). Ex-FIFA chief Jack Warner in UK court appeal against corruption charges. [online] Available at:
https://www.skysports.com/football/news/11095/11978212/ex-fifa-chief-jack-warner-in-uk-court-appeal-against-corruption-charges) [Accessed on 23 May 2020].

As it turns out, Dassler was the man who first created the broadcast and sponsorship rights model we know so well today but he needed the sports federations on board and that was where Havelange and Samaranch came in to form a very convenient friendship.

None of this was necessarily negative until you factored in the dirty tricks that took place behind the scenes as Dassler carefully moved his chess pieces to create a virtual ATM for himself. His new friends stood to gain too while the lion's share of the money, intended to go to the growth and development of the sports themselves, seldom trickled that far down.

Few would say sport was not better off with all the broadcast and sponsorship money pumped into it today. It helped make everything better but unfortunately, the benefits also extended to the bank balances of these villains. That would include their Swiss and Cayman Islands accounts by the way.

Not satisfied with the status quo, Italian Primo Nebiolo, who had risen to become president of the International Amateur Athletics Federation (IAAF) with the assistance of Dassler, teamed up with the German to create the World Athletics Championships in 1983.[8]

If you thought the first "A" in IAAF indicates that people did not get paid, well, you would be right but only as far as the athletes were concerned. Nebiolo, thanks to his German pal, was now also benefitting from broadcast and sponsorship money, just like Havelange and Samaranch.

These people had arranged additional money for themselves in the form of donations and commissions. Some people might prefer to call it bribery and kickbacks.

Whenever you see something suspicious in politics or public life, you would rightly question it. Why not do the same in sport? Did you know there is an organisation called the Association of National Olympic Committees (ANOC)? That is right.

There is an International Olympic Committee, which is a confederation of national Olympic committees, and now there is also the ANOC, a confederation of national Olympic committees. What is the point of ANOC's existence?

If you have not yet written your thesis, or if you are looking for a place to go investigate and maybe come up with a big scoop, go take a closer look at ANOC. I shall do you the courtesy of stepping aside and leaving it to you.

---

[8] Vyv Simson and Jennings, A. (1992). The lords of the rings: power, money and drugs in the modern Olympics. London: Simon & Schuster

These kinds of shenanigans are not only reserved for the elite international level. If anything, corruption is even more prevalent at a local level where a newshound reporter is unlikely to be sniffing around. Consider the National Lotto Distribution Agency in South Africa.

They were a division of the National Lottery responsible for distributing funds to charities, sport federations and so forth, as their name suggested. In 2013, SA Table Tennis was the grateful recipient of R8.2 million.[9] On 31 March 2015, it was reported that Volleyball South Africa (VSA) had received R3.2 million. This was despite Lottery grants for a federation being capped at R2 million.[10]

How did that happen? Well, it helped that the vice presidents of the South African Sports Confederation and Olympic Committee, or SASCOC, and SA Table Tennis were the same person; Hajera Kajee, who very conveniently also happened to be a former National Lotto Distribution Agency chairperson.[11]

As for Volleyball, it is a tiny sport by any measure in South Africa, much like table tennis, but then it couldn't harm VSA's cause that their former president, Tubby Reddy was also SASCOC's CEO at the time.

In another incredible story at an even more micro level, Boland Athletics, an Athletics South Africa (ASA) affiliate, received R1 million, the limit for provincial federations. The president of Boland Athletics is one Harold Adams, a man with two different national identification numbers; one for "Harold Adams" and another for his real name, "Jacob Herold Adams".

Adams was also a vice-president of ASA and served on the Sport and Recreation Distribution Agency of the National Lottery as its deputy chairperson. [12] Oh, and he was also a board member of the South African Institute of Drug Free Sport. Many hats and all that.

Interestingly, the William Lloyd Primary School in the Boland region received R720,000 from the National Lottery Distribution Trust Fund in a period where ASA and most of its provincial members received less. Pieter Lourens was the principal at William Lloyd and coincidentally was also the vice-president of Boland Athletics.[13] It paid to be a friend of Harold. Or was it Jacob Herald?

---

[9] Joffe, G. (2019). Sport: greed & betrayal. Independently Published. (p251)

[10] Joffe, G. (2019). Sport: greed & betrayal. Independently Published. (p259)

[11] Joffe, G. (2019). Sport: greed & betrayal. Independently Published. (p251)

[12] Joffe, G. (2019). Sport: greed & betrayal. Independently Published. (p86-87)

[13] Joffe, G. (2019). Sport: greed & betrayal. Independently Published. (p200)

It all made sense when you considered that the SASCOC president during this time was one Gideon Sam, the chairperson of the National Lotteries Distribution Trust Fund at the time when he won the SASCOC presidency in 2008.

This was exposed by the former CNN, SuperSport and 94.7 Highveld Stereo sports journalist, Graeme Joffe, who called it a "grave conflict of interests which made it easy to sway the votes of the numerous sporting federations who are dependent on Lottery funding".[14]

Joffe fell so foul of SASCOC, that he fled South Africa after receiving a phone call telling him his life was in danger. Joffe now lives in the United States.[15]

It is clear and obvious that sports administrators were not necessarily the nicest people around and that from the perspective of a journalist, they deserved to be treated the same way a current affairs reporter would treat a politician, or the way a business correspondent would handle a CEO.

After you have explained this to those questioning your choice to delve into sports journalism, you may still get the odd eye roll. After all, it was in the public interest if the president or prime minister of a country had been found guilty of corruption, but was it really in the public's interest if the head of a sports federation had been stealing money, or committed bribery?

Well, of course it is. Firstly theft, or money laundering, racketeering and the like, are all against the law in every country in the world as far as I am aware. Just because you are the chairman of everyone's favourite football team does not give you any special legal privileges.

Moreover, think about how much money supporters spend on team merchandise, match tickets, refreshments and other expenses (like travel) just to be able to attend games. Is it not in the interest of these people to know that their money has been subsidising criminal behaviour?

The reality was that many times these bad guys choose sports administration because they know that sports reporters are less likely to scrutinise them the way political reporters do. Do not feed their stereotype. Hold them accountable. Investigate, but remember that it is not just about the villains at boardroom level. Sometimes, our favourite players are the bad guys.

Pakistan cricketer, Mohammad Amir received money in 2010 to deliberately bowl illegal deliveries in a Test match against England. Amir was caught and

---

[14] Joffe, G. (2019). Sport: greed & betrayal. Independently Published. (p36)

[15] Joffe, G. (2019). Sport: greed & betrayal. Independently Published. (p196-205)

banned from the sport for five years.[16] South Africa's cricket captain from 1994–2000, Hansie Cronje was not as lucky.

Cronje was banned for life after being involved in a match-fixing scheme in which he deliberately conspired to lose matches in exchange for money and other gifts from bookmakers.[17]

But beware. Some of your fellow sports journalists might not be as keen to investigate. In some cases, it might simply not be their beat. That is not a negative thing. Some sports journalists will work exclusively in an area where it is virtually impossible to investigate or break news.

For example, a desk producer at a television news channel is more likely to get a high-quality match highlights package on air than breaking the Cronje story. If you chose to be the desk producer, or any other type of softer journalism, then this book is still for you, so fret not.

In a later chapter, I shall share with you how you can still be close to the action even without being an investigative reporter. The point of this chapter is to illustrate to you that there are people getting away with proverbial murder in sport and they needed to be held accountable.

You do not have to be a hard-hitting reporter but please, do not be a "fan with a laptop". When you work in journalism, you need to keep your personal feelings to yourself. If you want to cheer, then do so in private. You do not want to be the sports reporter who high-fives a colleague in the press area of a stadium after the home team scores a try, as I witnessed at a Super 14 rugby match in Johannesburg in 2009.

Cycling fans did not want to believe that American Lance Armstrong could have cheated his way to winning seven straight Tour de France titles. [18] Hansie

---

[16] ESPN cricinfo. (n.d.). Mohammad Amir profile and biography, stats, records, averages, photos and videos. [online] Available at: https://www.espncricinfo.com/pakistan/content/player/290948.html [Accessed 23 May 2020]

[17] ESPNcricinfo. (n.d.). Hansie Cronje profile and biography, stats, records, averages, photos and videos. [online] Available at: https://www.espncricinfo.com/southafrica/content/player/44485.html [Accessed 23 May 2020]

[18] published, C.S. (2021). Lance Armstrong | Cycling Weekly. [online] cyclingweekly.com. Available at: https://www.cyclingweekly.com/tag/lance-armstrong [Accessed 23 May 2020].

Cronje's supporters did not want to believe that he was guilty either. That is fine if you are a diehard fan, but the journalists cannot simply decide that someone is innocent or guilty based on nothing other than their personal feelings.

Sadly, there were many cycling journalists who refused to believe that Armstrong could be guilty of doping. They had already celebrated him as one of the great cyclists of all-time and just like Tiger Woods in golf, and Roger Federer in tennis, Armstrong had become the face of the sport. The American had become a global icon and in the case of many reporters, a personal favourite.

Do not forget, this guy had beaten cancer before going on that phenomenal hot streak. Unfortunately, we now know that Armstrong was a drugs cheat and the official record now shows that from 1999 to 2005, there was no winner of the Tour de France.

David Walsh was the journalist who exposed Armstrong but he was met with much resistance, sadly from his fellow professionals, but Walsh persisted and in the end Armstrong, who once referred to Walsh as the "little troll", was outed as a drugs cheat. Walsh's work is an example of journalism excellence.[19] It goes without saying that Walsh's pursuit of the truth managed to get under Armstrong's skin.

The late Andrew Jennings was the journalist who exposed the irregularities at the International Olympic Committee (IOC) and FIFA, and became the first journalist ever to be banned from FIFA press conferences in 2003 after famously asking the organisation's president, 'Herr Blatter, have you ever taken a bribe?'

Notice how in both instances, the journalist who was working hard to expose the truth was vilified by those in influential or powerful positions. This should come as no surprise. You do not have to be the kind of reporter who sends shudders downthe spines of sporting federation board members, but it is not a bad reputation to have in this business.

I would recommend you get your hands on *Undercover Reporting*. Of particular interest is the chapter *Crusaders And Zealots*. The book deals with the truth about deception and by now, you can see why this was important.

Brooke Kroeger wrote that almost no clandestine group had escaped the disloyal scrutiny of infiltrators who gained access to its secrets and then shared

---

[19] the Guardian. (2014). How I brought down drug-taking Lance Armstrong, by David Walsh. [online] Available at:
https://www.theguardian.com/media/greenslade/2014/jan/28/lance-armstrong-sundaytimes.

them for publication against the organisation's wishes. In years gone by, journalists had used deceptive tactics to penetrate these and other secretive societies, religious groups, and so forth.

This was often done to frame the reporting in graphic storybook details, in classic journalistic "show" rather than "tell". On other occasions, the ploy's purpose was to verify information that would be difficult if not impossible to obtain otherwise.[20]

Now obviously, FIFA or the IOC are not clandestine organisations, but if you dug a little deeper, you would find that there was plenty of secretive activity and the first question had to be "Why?"

I don't suggest you resort to cloak-and-dagger tactics to uncover information, but I want you to consider the way journalists in days of yore had gone about gathering information to break stories. Think about how you might have gone about exposing Jack Warner, for example.

Now that you have justified why sport deserves journalism, it is time to look at just how big a deal sport is. One of the key reasons, as you may have detected by now, is because it attracts villains. Why does it attract these people? Money. There is big money in sport.

I want to present you with some numbers of the nosebleed variety, courtesy of fintech start up, Qara. According to research done by A.T. Kearney[21], the global sports market is worth somewhere between $480 billion and $620 billion with a compound annual growth rate (CAGR) of 5.9%.

The USA has the biggest market sector so far, amounting to $31.83 billion. The sports industry is the second-fastest growing sector for brands, outpacing the GDP growth of most countries. The sports industry in America was projected to reach $75 billion in 2019.

Did you get that? The sports industry is a sector so big that it is bigger than some countries. Imagine the president or prime minister of your country going to Dallas Cowboys owner, Jerry Jones and asking for a loan, or approaching the president of FC Barcelona, Joan Laporta, requesting investment.

---

[20] Kroeger, B. and Hamill, P. (2012). CRUSADERS AND ZEALOTS. [online] JSTOR. Available at: http://www.jstor.org/stable/j.ctt22727sf.16 [Accessed 24 May 2020]. (pp. 209-210)

[21] QARA (2019). Sports Industry Insights. [online] Medium. Available at: https://medium.com/qara/sports-industry-report-3244bd253b8.

Feel free to point that out to your peers who have been sniffing around Meta, Amazon, Apple, Netflix or Alphabet for a scoop. Why not go see what the local sports franchise is up to? Believe me, there is a story there.

The numbers extend to the sports analytics market, which was valued at $56 million in 2018. In 2018, sports sponsorship revenue in North America amounted to $17 billion. According to a report by the Association of Summer Olympic International Federations, also known by the acronym ASOIF, (more on them later), global sponsorship of sport stood at $66 billion, leading the way ahead of gate and media rights revenues (both at $46.8 billion) and then merchandising at $20.8 billion.[22]

The National Football League (NFL) is by far the most successful American sports league in history. Bloomberg estimated that the NFL earned nearly $15 billion in 2018. And Statista revealed that more than 50% of the league's revenue came from TV deals. Compare this to the English Premier League, which according to the Deloitte Sports Business Group had revenue amounting to $6.1 billion for the 2017/2018 season, up 6% from its previous year.

That was the kind of money that should get attention from someone like Richard Quest on CNN, right? Well, Richard is more concerned with traditional businesses and what they were up to. There is nothing wrong with that. That is Richard's beat. Perhaps your beat could be following the money in sport.

In sports business, sponsorship is everything. It drives profits, provides funds, and allows for competitive events to be run. PwC had reported that the sponsorship market would reach $49 billion by 2023. While sponsorship was important for many sports organisations, consumers had criticised corporate presence taking away the purity in sports competition; thereby making sport all about profits. Those people lost the argument a very long time ago.

Media rights are essentially the fees that customers have to pay to watch sports on TV, the internet, or any other media distribution channel. Media rights were expected to reach $23.8 billion in revenue in 2022 and represented nearly 30% of all sports revenues.

The biggest players behind media rights came from tech giants like Meta, Amazon, Apple, Netflix and Alphabet. If you just thought that you read those five

---

[22] FUTURE OF GLOBAL SPORT ASSOCIATION OF SUMMER OLYMPIC INTERNATIONAL FEDERATIONS.
(2019). [online] Available at:
https://www.asoif.com/sites/default/files/download/future_of_global_sport.pdf.

names just a few paragraphs ago, you would be quite right. Keep reading for more on that quintet and its interest in sport.

As sports businesses continued to grow, venture investing was becoming more popular with institutional and retail investors. Since 2012, investments for start-ups related to sports had grown nearly 30% each year. In 2015 alone, nearly $1 billion was invested in sport-tech start-ups. Investors were actively looking for disruptive and innovative technologies to boost businesses in the sports industry.

According to Sport Marketing Quarterly[23], when marketers began to use television as an advertising tool, ad revenue immediately grew tenfold, from $12.3 million in 1949 to $128 million in 1951. Web advertising revenue grew at a greater rate during a similar period of development from $55 million in 1995 to $900 million in 1997.[24]

Let us look at television, media and sponsorship money and it would become very clear, very quickly, why an administrator (or politician keen to avoid the scrutiny of hard-core investigative reporters) would be attracted to sport, and similarly, why you as a sports journalist should be attracted to finding out their true motives.

In my home country of South Africa, MultiChoice acquired the television broadcast rights to South Africa's leading domestic football competition, the Premier Soccer League (PSL) in 2007. The five-year deal was worth R1.6 billion, around three times the value of the PSL's previous contract with the South African Broadcasting Corporation (SABC).[25] At the time, one U.S. dollar was worth about R6.95, so in those days that would have been a shade over $230 million.

One of the controversies around that deal was that it shifted the local football league from terrestrial television to a satellite subscription service, meaning many of the country's football fans were likely to miss out. South Africa is a country that has high unemployment numbers and high levels of poverty. The majority of citizens cannot afford the satellite service.

---

[23] Anon, (n.d.). [online] Available at: http://www.measure4you.de/images/AnalysisOfOnlineMarketingInTheSportsIndustry.pdf.

[24] Fosket, S. (1996, November). Online technology ushers in one-to-one market. *Direct Marketing.* 59(7), 38-40

[25] Shandu, K. 2008. The Business of Soccer and Television-What's In It? Journal of Marketing, February/March, pp. 65–79

Contrastingly, it was a great deal for the PSL, whose board members had negotiated a deal that would swell the organisation's coffers. That money would also naturally trickle down to the clubs and ensure higher salaries for the players as well as giving clubs the ability to invest and reinvest in their facilities. As you can see, there were pros and cons to these broadcast and sponsorship deals.

The PSL's board members did indeed dole out commissions to themselves but by the first decade of the 21st century that had largely become the norm. You may argue that the likes of Havelange, Samaranch and Dassler set the precedent. The PSL does actually hand out monthly grants to clubs in the Premiership and the second tier Championship, and by most accounts without these grants, the Championship clubs would likely face a daily struggle against foreclosure. That broadcast rights money made it possible to survive.

In the United Kingdom, the partial delisting of English Test cricket led to a significant increase in the annual broadcast revenues for the English Cricket Board from £15 million between 1995 and 1998, when it was available on free-to-air, to over £50 million between 2006 and 2009 when home Test matches were on the satellite platform.[26]

When we deal with the English Premier League, the numbers become even bigger. The financial crisis of 2008 and subsequent austerity of many European nations did not prevent the value of rights to the Premier League rising from £1.6 billion in 2011 to £3 billion in 2014 and £5.1 billion from 2016.[27]

There is no question that the Premier League is the top dog in European football but it was in fact, a Spanish club that is top of the Money League published by Deloitte,[28] considered the most contemporary and reliable independent analysis of the clubs' relative financial performance.

---

[26] DCMS (2009). Review of Free-to-air Listed Events Report by the Independent Advisory Panel to the Secretary of State for Culture, Media and Sport. [online] Available at: http://webarchive.nationalarchives.gov.uk/+/http:/www.culture.gov.uk/images/consultations/indep endentpanelreport-to-SoS-Free-to-air-Nov2009.pdf [Accessed 4 November 2018].

[27] Gemmell, J. (2018). BBC Sport in Black and White, by Richard Haynes. The International Journal of the History of Sport, 35(11), pp.1209–1211.

[28] Deloitte (2021). Deloitte Football Money League | Deloitte UK. [online] Deloitte United Kingdom. Available at: https://www2.deloitte.com/uk/en/pages/sports-business-group/articles/deloitte-football-money-league.html.

Published just eight months after the end of the 2018/19 season, FC Barcelona reached the top of the Money League for the first time and at the same time, became the first club to break the €800 million barrier, generating revenue of €840.8 million.

The top 20 highest earning football clubs for the 2018/19 season had combined revenues of €9.3 billion – up 11%. Did your salary increase by 11% in the last financial year?

Italian Serie A club Juventus FC rounds up the top 10 but that could be set to change with an injection of additional revenue that we shall discuss later in this chapter.

According to a 2019 Deloitte Annual Review of Football Finance29, the German Bundesliga's new four-year media rights arrangements contributed to an uplift of €290 million in broadcast revenues, while the return of Stuttgart and Hannover 96 to Germany's top flight, at the expense of Darmstadt and Inglostadt, for the 2017/18 season helped to deliver a boost to attendances, and subsequently match day revenues, which increased 7% to €538 million, after falling in the previous season.

These promoted clubs, along with the likes of Schalke 04 and Eintracht Frankfurt, played key roles in the league, achieving steady revenue growth of 4% relating to sponsorship and other commercial activities.

You do not have to be a genius to figure out how disastrous it would be for these top leagues if their most popular teams suddenly started to struggle. Clearly, it was in the Bundesliga's interest to have Bayern Munich winning, or to have Stuttgart and Hannover 96 in their league rather than Darmstadt and Inglostadt.

Meanwhile, Real Madrid's success in European competition, and Barcelona's new four-year shirt front sponsorship with Rakuten, drove the Spanish league's commercial revenue growth by 14%, as these powerhouse clubs formed a Spanish one-two at the top of the 2019 Deloitte Football Money League.

Barca and Real Madrid's success trickled down to the coffers of Spain's La Liga. Who said trickle-down economics was not effective? What this meant was that these leagues were never going to do anything to jeopardise the potential for

---

29 https://www2.deloitte.com/content/dam/Deloitte/uk/Documents/sports-business-group/deloitte-uk-annual-review-of-football-finance-2019.pdf (Michael Barnard, Sam Boor, Christopher Winn, Chris Wood and Izzy Wray)

their most popular (read top revenue generators) to be successful. The days of a small village team punching above their weight and rising all the way to the top division before challenging for the big trophies live firmly in the 20th century.

A great story for an investigative sports reporter to track would be the sustainability of these models. Paris Saint-Germain was able to spend a world record transfer fee of €222 million to sign Brazilian forward Neymar, but no club has a black hole budget.

Now in the modern context, PSG could afford this transfer fee but what about wages? According to the Deloitte report, the wages-to-revenue ratio across the "big five" (England, Spain, Italy, Germany and France) increased to 62% as wages spending outpaced revenue growth, increasing by 13% to total over €9 billion for the first time.

English Premier League clubs continued to spend the additional revenues received from the last broadcast cycle, which commenced in 2016/17, with wage costs increasing by 15% to almost £2.9 billion. This increase pushed Europe's biggest spending league to a wages-to-revenue ratio of 59%, and with lower growth projections for future revenue, this was likely to return above 60% and remain there for the foreseeable future.

2017/18 saw French Ligue 1 clubs' wage costs increase rapidly, up 17% on 2016/17, as a high-level of receipts from transfers, the impact of recent investment at several clubs and the security of agreed broadcast revenue uplifts from 2018/19, and more significantly, from 2020/21, gave clubs the opportunity to boost wages spending on new talent.

Olympique Marseille's wage bill increased by 43% to over €125 million, while PSG's wage costs increase of €60 million contributed around a third of overall growth, due to the high-profile acquisitions of Neymar and Kylian Mbappé.

AS Monaco also increased their spending by over 30% as these three clubs together accounted for over 70% of the leagues' additional cost. Worryingly, this saw the average wages-to-revenue ratio increase by nine percentage points to 75%; in excess of the 70% ratio often considered to be a benchmark for sustainability.

Manchester United (£296 million) continued to be the Premier League's highest wage payers, but while wages increased by more than £30 million, the club continued to have a relatively favourable wages-to-revenue ratio (50%). Only two clubs recorded a wages-to-revenue ratio of less than 50% in 2017/18.

Promoted club Huddersfield Town spent the least (£63 million) and were rewarded for showing relative restraint as they narrowly avoided relegation to the second-tier Championship. Tottenham Hotspur (39%) became only the third club to spend less than 40% of its revenue on wages since 1998/99, and this was not detrimental to on-pitch performance as the club qualified for the Champions League once again, and subsequently reached the final.

Eight Premier League clubs reported a wages-to-revenue ratio in excess of the 70%. This represented a considerable increase on the previous season in which only two clubs reported a ratio above this threshold and perhaps unsurprisingly, in the 2017/18 season, six of the seven highest wage spenders finished in the top seven places.

Earlier, I mentioned that leagues would not want their most popular teams to struggle or, worse, suffer relegation. In 2016/17, Newcastle United (home stadium capacity of approximately 52 000) and Aston Villa (home stadium capacity of approximately 42 000) were playing in the Championship. That was not ideal for the Premier League.

In order to help teams that had been relegated, the Premier League supplied these teams with so-called parachute payments. Over a three-year period, clubs received an annual bonus from the Premier League to help them combat the financial losses of not being in the top division and at the same time, aid their challenge in securing a swift promotion back to the top-tier.

Parachute payments created financial polarisation among the Championship clubs. The revenue gap went beyond the division and was increasing both from the top of the Championship to the bottom of the Premier League and from the bottom of the Championship to the top of League One (third-tier).

The gap between the average revenue for a relegated Premier League club and a promoted Championship club had increased from £43 million in 2012/13 to £94 million in 2017/18, while the gap between the average wage bill for a relegated Championship club and promoted League One club had increased from £13 million to £21 million across the same period.

This potentially made it more challenging for promoted clubs to become established in the Premier League and Championship without further investment.

The new Premier League broadcast rights cycle started in the 2019/20 season, and the value of broadcast distributions to clubs had remained reasonably static with parachute payments not seeing any significant growth. Gaining promotion to the Premier League would generate a revenue uplift similar to the 2017/18 season of at least £170 million, based on Premier League distributions and guaranteed parachute payments if relegated, rising to at least £300 million if the promoted clubs survive more than one season.

Parachute payments, in respect of recent relegation from the Premier League accounted for 32% of total revenue in 2017/18 in the Championship. Eight Championship clubs were in receipt of parachute payments, ranging from £17 million to £42 million, totalling £243 million, the highest total amount ever paid in a single season.

Aston Villa had the highest wage costs in the Championship in 2017/18 of £73 million, more than seven times that of Burton Albion (who recorded the lowest wages spend, at just under £10 million). Aston Villa's wages bill was the third-highest ever recorded in the Championship, behind Newcastle United's £112 million in 2016/17 and Queens Park Rangers' £75 million in 2013/14. The average wages spend per club was £33 million, an increase from £30 million in 2016/17

Excluding Newcastle United, the wages-to-revenue ratio was 95% in 2016/17, a tentative indication that the Championship could be home to several clubs who were one bad decision away from financial ruin. The situation worsened just one season later.

2017/18 saw a wages-to-revenue ratio of 106% as clubs continued to increase wage spend in the quest to win promotion. Cardiff City had the sixth-highest wage spend in 2017/18 as it gained automatic promotion to the Premier League, while also disclosing £23 million in bonuses and other commitments due following promotion.

Was this sustainable? Who needed to be held accountable? You are in investigative reporter territory right now and best of all, your business journalist colleagues were unlikely to cover this. Maybe this could be your niche.

Interestingly, changes of ownership were more prevalent among English football clubs than in any other European market. There have been over 50 changes of majority ownership among Premier League and Championship clubs since 2005. Contributing to this churn, English football attracted more foreign interest than elsewhere.

At the end of the 2018/19 season, around 60% of clubs in the top two divisions had a foreign owner. The attraction for investors was the Premier Leagues' multi-billion broadcast rights arrangements, a key driver for investors' interest.

As of 2019/20, these rights would generate around £3 billion per season for the Premier League. Not only did these rights deliver substantial and secure annual revenue for clubs, they also gave access to a global television audience eager to watch the star clubs and players competing for ten months each year in what many consider to be "the world's most exciting league".

For some owners, matches broadcast to one billion homes across 190 countries provided a global opportunity that could be exploited through new marketing and commercial arrangements. For others, owning such a trophy asset provided them with useful media and business exposure, access to important corporate, personal and political relationships, and excitement and emotional returns if on-pitch results went well.

With all Premier League clubs ranking in the world's top 40 for club revenues, they were economically strong participants in the global transfer market to sign some of the world's top football stars and, at the top end, capable of competing strongly in UEFA club competitions.

Imagine owning or running one of these top revenue-generating clubs and sharing in its profits. You could be the highest or one of the highest paid sports administrators on Earth. Or you could just be Cristiano Ronaldo.

In 2018, Ronaldo changed clubs. Juventus paid Real Madrid €117 million for the then-33-year old. That in itself was almost unthinkable. Many questioned the wisdom of signing an older player for such a high fee. Before we look at the benefits for the Italian club, let us look at the team's outlay just on Ronaldo as per a KPMG report.[30]

The Portuguese player's reported salary was €30 million; gross cost of approximately €55–56 million on the part of Juve, representing 21% of the club's total staff costs.

How could Juventus protect its asset against any unforeseeable negative event? There were principally three types of insurance programmes and risk transfer solutions that specialised Sports Personal Accident insurers provide football clubs with:

---

[30] Ronal do Economi cs. (n.d.). [online] Available at:
https://www.footballbenchmark.com/documents/files/public/KPMG%20Football%20B enchmark_Ronaldo%20Economics(1).pdf

1. Accidental Death (AD) and Permanent Total Disability (PTD), usually offered in combination.
2. Life, generally the least expensive and most traditional insurance, covering naturally caused death, which was mainly driven by the player's age and pre-existing medical and current health conditions.
3. Temporary Total Disability (TTD), also called salary or income protection.

Total annual insurance costs for Ronaldo were estimated to cost the club between €3 and 5 million.

Juventus FC tended to enjoy good home support, so it was not as if the Ronaldo signing would have a dramatic increase in ticket sales but season ticket prices for the 2018/19 Serie A season did increase at an average of approximately 30% on the previous season's pricing.

Thus, if the total number of season ticket subscribers remained the same as the previous year (29 300), Juventus would generate €33–34 million from this source (compared to €24 million for 2016/17). In addition to match day revenues for Serie A games, Juve could also enjoy higher receipts for hosting UEFA Champions League matches.

Within three football seasons, KPMG believed it was realistic for the Turin club to add an additional €75–100 million. The club would also be able to increase the international portfolio of their sponsors, targeting those countries where their brand was less popular.

More than 40% of Juve's sponsors were Italy-based, with relatively few regional partners in Asia, North America and Africa. On the other hand, clubs like Manchester United, Real Madrid and Barcelona had only between 15% and 25% local sponsors.

In the 2015/16 season, Juventus FC switched their kit supplier from Nike to Adidas for €139.5 million for six seasons. This made for an average annual value of €23.25 million, representing an increase of 88% compared to their earlier agreement with the American sportswear giant.

In the new agreement, the club decided to manage merchandising and licencing activities on their own, giving up on the fixed basis of €6 million originally agreed upon with the technical sponsor. Such strategy had already paid some dividends, as in the 2016/17 season, the club recorded €19.2 million from this source.

Obviously, the arrival of Cristiano Ronaldo represented a clear opportunity to increase merchandising, especially considering the sale of his jersey, as well as that of other players, and hopefully bringing a boost to international popularity for Juventus.

It would appear as if the ostensibly outlandish fee spent on Ronaldo was easily justifiable for Juve; commercially at least. Now just imagine if Juventus had actually won the Champions League while Ronaldo was at the club. We shall never know as he transferred to Manchester United in 2021.

Nevertheless, the Portuguese superstar represented a company in and of himself, thanks to massive media reach. He is known throughout the world in part thanks to his massive numbers on the main social media platforms: Facebook, Instagram and Twitter (comprising 841 million followers in total at the time of writing). Follower numbers for an athlete like LeBron James, or for a pop star like Justin Bieber (230 million and 655 million, respectively) fall short in comparison.

Such massive visibility does not go unnoticed for his sponsors, who were willing to remunerate him between €350 000 and €500 000 per Instagram post, ranking him as the most profitable athlete worldwide in such terms.

He had about four times as many followers as Juventus at the time of signing. Compared to current employer, Al-Nassr (the Saudi club he joined in 2022), he comfortably outnumbered them too. Unsurprisingly, before even stepping on the pitch with a black and white jersey, the acquisition of Ronaldo resulted in high visibility for Juve, with social media numbers already headed upward.

Indeed, if a star player like Ronaldo moved to a new team, he also brought his sizeable follower base with him, as, to a certain extent, fans tend to link more with individuals than clubs these days. Consider the figures for Juventus FC official accounts on Facebook, Instagram and Twitter from 5th July to 17th July 2018. There was an uptick of between 15% and 25% in follower numbers. This could be called the "Cristiano Ronaldo effect".

Earlier, you read about Barcelona's position at the top of the football tree. Well that did not last as long as they would have liked. Fierce rivals Real Madrid were the world's most valuable club, according to the Brand Finance Football 50 2021 report[31].

[31] Anon, (n.d.). Messi's Departure Could Cost Barcelona €137 Million in Brand Value | Press Release | Brand Finance. [online] Available at: https://brandfinance.com/press-releases/messi-departure-could-cost-barcelona-137-million-in-brand-value.

Barca would not be helped by the departure of Lionel Messi to Paris Saint-Germain. The report estimated that this transfer could devalue Barcelona by as much as 11%, knocking off €137 million in the process. Messi's departure was expected to have directly negative effects on the club's future sponsorship income, merchandise sales and match day revenue, not to mention a decline in brand value.

Back to Ronaldo. The positive aspects were there for all to see but by now, you must have worked out that it was also a breeding ground for all kinds of unscrupulous behaviour. You could just picture some dodgy character with an even dodgier business model, clamouring to get Ronaldo to promote his product.

Was Ronaldo vulnerable to this? Had he sufficiently safeguarded himself with trustworthy people who act as gatekeepers to the football star? Or were they in on the act, receiving a kickback in return for delivering an appearance from Ronaldo?

The football superstar had faced legal battles on accusations of tax evasion in Spain and a rape charge in Las Vegas and while those were issues of enormous seriousness, there was no known social media-related controversy surrounding the Portuguese.

But have other young, exciting footballers, who suddenly find themselves the flavour of the week, been as careful? Who said sports journalism was not a serious business?

While we are still on the topic of football, consider the 2018 FIFA World Cup in Russia. Despite what the IOC would like to believe, football's world cup is the biggest sporting event in the world. A Nielson report[32] documents that more than 3.5 billion people watched the event while 1.12 billion watched the final. Imagine the kind of revenue that was generated from advertising and sponsorship.

This chapter has hitherto tried hard to point out that many of the positives in sport were exploited by crooks, and that that is a great place for an aspiring investigative sports reporter to focus, but it was not always bad news. The city of Sochi received more tourists during the 2018 World Cup than its actual population.

Imagine what that did for the local economy. According to the Nielsen report, the fans who visited Sochi for the football, also spent time and money in other areas, some more predictable than others like:

---

[32] http://nielsensports.com/wp-content/uploads/2014/09/FIFAReport-2018.pdf

- 68% visited bars, cafes and restaurants.
- 38% toured the city.
- 32% visited museums, galleries or cultural venues.
- 21% went shopping.
- 15% attended local music festivals, cultural shows, or concerts.

FIFA's official fan parks were called fan fests and the tournament's official mascot, the bear Zabivaka, registered more than 40 000 plush toy sales at fan fests and 51% of those who purchased official merchandise also purchased the official mascot plush toy. Ask your marketing friends about upselling.

It appears that many football fans do not care too much about the Blatters and Warners of this world, or do not know enough about their villainy, since globally, 53% of fans were likely to purchase products from FIFA's official sponsors and 61% say they would be proud to work for a company that sponsored the World Cup.

Given what you know about Horst Dassler, would you be proud to work at Adidas, or would you be you satisfied the shoe and apparel manufacturer has put that seedy bit of history behind it? Mind you, would it be important to you at all?

Have you heard of the FAANG stocks? Of course you have. You have already read about them twice just in this chapter. Still unclear? Ask your friend who intends to go into business reporting. If they do not know, suggest they study something else.

In the animal kingdom, the Big Five consists of the lion, rhino, elephant, buffalo and leopard in Africa. The stock market version of the Big Five is the FAANG stocks: Facebook (Meta), Amazon, Apple, Netflix and Google (or Alphabet as the parent company is known).

These blue-chip stocks are of such value and offer their investors such growth that they had been grouped together as a super stocks quintet. These five companies were disruptors and innovators. If you wanted to know in which direction the world was headed, it is possible that one of these tech giants was leading the way there.

With that in mind, did you know that tech giants were getting into sport? Sorry, correction, they are already there. You can watch NFL matches on Twitter, Amazon Prime has its own Premier League deal and there are already sports matches being broadcast on Facebook. I tell you this because while the innovation was great, it also opened an opportunity for a villain. The exact kind of villain that a good reporter would expose. Think about that.

Speaking of villains, traditionally the stereotype has not been kind to bookmakers. Have you noticed how many sports teams, especially in football, have betting companies as their shirt sponsors? Now, it would be wrong of us to simply assume that there was skulduggery taking place, but it would not be beyond anyone's imagination to see trouble brewing.

International sports betting is estimated to have a market capitalisation of $250 billion; 50% of U.S. citizens had reportedly admitted to betting in sport events and therefore, it made sense for bookmakers to get in there, as per a Qara report.[33]

The report stated that in 2016, the sports betting market in the U.S. was valued at $40 billion. Research also showed that due to new technologies and digital connectivity, the market is expected to surge in the near future. It would be interesting to see what happens with this industry that is largely considered to be a social evil. Already in England the Premier League has taken action. In April 2023 it was announced its clubs have collectively agreed to withdraw gambling sponsorship from the front of their matchday shirts by the end of the 2025/26 season.

It is debatable how much of an impact that will make given that the clubs will still be able to feature gambling brands on their shirt sleeves as well as LED advertising inside the stadiums. At the time of writing, eight Premier League clubs have gambling companies on the front of their shirts, worth an estimated £60 million per year. The English Football League which is responsible for the next three leagues in the country's pyramid is currently sponsored by Sky Bet and has made no moves to curtail betting sponsorship at the time of writing.[34]

A few decades ago, cigarette and alcohol brands were the key sponsors in sport. Cricket fans of a certain generation may even fondly recall that there was a time when every other tournament was called the *Benson & Hedges Series*.

---

[33] QARA (2019). Sports Industry Insights. [online] Medium. Available at: https://medium.com/qara/sports-industry-report-3244bd253b8

[34] BBC Sport. (2021, January 8). Premier League clubs agree to trial concussion substitutes and additional permanent substitutions. BBC News. Retrieved from https://www.bbc.com/sport/football/65260002#:~:text=Premier%20League%20clubs% 20have%20collectively,shirt%20sleeves%20and%20LED%20advertising.

Cigarette and alcohol advertising are now banned in enough parts of the world for these companies to not even bother.

There was a time when the famous South African beer, Castle Lager, sponsored the country's national rugby team. However, when the Springboks were in action away from home in Europe, they could not display Castle Lager on their shirts, so instead went with the alternative "Charles", in reference to the beer's founder, Charles Glass.

The gimmick extended to other sports too. Benson & Hedges sponsored the Jordan Formula One team and used the alternative "Buzzin' Hornets" at one stage. Rothmans was instead "R.?" on the Williams car. It was never going to last though. How long would we see bookmakers on our favourite team's shirts before politicians begin to think of it as a bad influence on society?

Perhaps not long at all if you consider the following story. Popular Wigan Athletic Football Club owner Dave Whelan sold the club to International Entertainment Corporation (IEC) in 2018, controlled by Hong Kong businessman Stanley Choi Chiu-fai, a keen poker player who in 2012 won HK$50 million at the Macau High Stakes Challenge.

IEC was an investment holding company whose activities and interests included hotels and property leasing of casinos, leisure and entertainment operations. The word "casinos" should have caught your attention.

Choi would then sell the club to the Next Leader Fund (NLF), a Hong Kong-based consortium registered in the Cayman Islands, on 29 May 2020. Choi also had a 51% controlling interest with fellow Hong Kong businessman, Au Yeung Wai Kay holding the remaining 49%.

Choi had effectively sold the club to himself. He then quit in June, prompted by business issues in The Philippines, leaving Au Yeung in charge with reports he had paid £40 million for the club.

According to The Press and Journal, on 1st July at 06:00 the next morning, an email was circulated, stating the club had been put into administration. Au Yeung blamed Covid-19, the inability to sell season tickets and Britain's exit from the European Union. The English Football League (EFL) was not convinced.

The club had 12 league table points deducted, which virtually condemned them to relegation to the third-tier of English football.35 Wigan unsuccessfully appealed the deduction and were ultimately relegated.

But what of Choi? There was video of EFL chairman, Rick Parry discussing a bet placed in The Philippines that the club would be relegated. The Philippines was where Choi happened to have gambling interests. IEC was involved in the casino business, remember. Did Choi effectively sell the club to himself, and then in his capacity as previous owner bet on the club to be relegated, while knowing in his capacity as current owner that a points-deduction penalty was on the cards making relegation a certainty?

Even though the bet had been dismissed as a red herring, these were serious allegations and the supporters of Wigan Athletic, who got together and crowdfunded more than £150,000 to help their team travel to an away game against Barnsley that July, deserved to know the truth.

The United Nations' *Transnational Organized Crime in Southeast Asia: Evolution, Growth and Impact 2019* report said, "The region's rapidly expanding network of casinos, many of which are lightly or not at all regulated, has emerged as a perfect partner or offshoot industry for organized crime groups that need to launder large volumes of illicit money". For additional fuel to this fire, Wigan also just happened to be sponsored by KB88, an online betting company based in The Philippines.[36]

Who was it again that said sport was not important or serious?

In 2003, World Wrestling Entertainment (WWE) visited South Africa. My dad and I went to the show at the Good Hope Centre in Cape Town. It was a fun and entertaining event and no one could turn around and accuse WWE of not putting on an excellent show.

---

[35] Durent, J. (n.d.). Kevin McNaughton reveals shock and sympathy at Wigan Athletic plight as club highlights financial and ownership shortcomings of Championship life. [online] Press and Journal. Available at:
https://www.pressandjournal.co.uk/fp/sport/football/2327207/2327207/ [Accessed 25 May 2020].

[36] South China Morning Post. (2020). Finger-pointing, the Philippines and EFL-what happened at Wigan? [online] Available at:
https://www.scmp.com/sport/football/article/3092949/wigan-athletic-and-hong-kong-based-mystery-finger-pointing [Accessed 25 May 2020].

The fact remained though that professional wrestling is not a sport, it is entertainment. Some who turn their noses up at professional wrestling may even point out that it is nothing but a soap opera, and they would be right. Is professional wrestling a sport? No, it is not but what about eSports? Is gaming a sport? This is something that divides opinions.

Perhaps you were of the persuasion that gaming is nothing but a recreational activity and deserves no space at all in the sports section of a news bulletin? You may well be right but just like other activities that divides opinion on whether or not they are actually sports, like snooker, pool, darts and chess, it is beginning to demand attention, if not respect.

Revenues for eSports reached $1.1 billion in 2019 and during the 2020 Covid-19 pandemic where almost every country on Earth was under a lockdown of some variety, eSports was the go-to for many traditional sports. For example, real-life Formula One drivers took part in an eSports Formula One grand prix. Could this be a sign of things to come?

Whether you like it or not, eSports is now a thing and you could very well find yourself working at a media house where the editor has been converted to the lure of eSports. That means your first assignment could be to go cover the local, regional, national or even international eSports Championships.

This particular sector has grown tremendously over the past couple of years. With an increase in viewership as well as its revenue, Newzoo estimated that the annual growth rate for eSports would reach approximately 14%.

Regardless of how you personally view eSports, you had best get used to it. Oh, and since revenues have now surpassed the billion-dollar mark, you might want to pay attention to who the people are that are running eSports. Who are they? How did they get there? Why are they there? What are their intentions? Where is all the money going?

According to Deloitte's *2020 Sports Industry Outlook* prepared by Pete Giorgio, Activision Blizzard, Riot and Valve are the current leaders in the eSports industry, but the ecosystem is expanding. Keep an eye out on platforms such as Twitch, YouTube Gaming, Facebook Gaming, Mixer, and Smashcast; Huya, Douya, and PandaTV in China; and OGN in South Korea, in addition to more integrated sponsorships that can occur in-game and as part of eSports events.

Also keep an eye out on eSports players and personalities like Ninja and DrLupo who could become more mainstream and more players than ever could secure opportunities to work with endemic and non-endemic brands looking for ways to influence hard-to-reach audiences.

Furthermore, you might want to keep an eye on the rise of cryptocurrencies and non-fungible tokens (NFTs). Still in its infancy, it is possible to make in-game purchases now with NFTs. These tokens are all backed by a cryptocurrency, like Ethereum or Solana, for example.

Some say this is an early peak at what Mark Zuckerberg's metaverse might look like. Perhaps but you just know there is a villain lurking looking to exploit an opportunity. Be vigilant, young investigative reporter.

Another area where sport is experiencing significant growth is in the area of women's sport. According to Deloitte, many companies now view women's sports as a powerful diversity and inclusion platform. The momentum around women's sports has also opened unparalleled opportunities for the creation of new professional leagues, franchises, corporate sponsorships, and increased ticket sales.

However, women's sport continues to have some challenges, including smaller prize pools, lower overall attendance, less attractive broadcast exposure, and fewer sponsorship dollars.

Nevertheless, Deloitte said with an even brighter spotlight on women's sports, sports organisations should consider doubling down on their investments. This could drive growth that not only benefitted leagues and franchises, but female athletes as well.

Sponsors should consider getting involved now to capitalise on the new opportunities and avenues for engagement that this growth area may create. Broadcasters could drive overall interest in women's sport by contributing to the value of current deals and together with sponsors, support year-round women's sports by leveraging the momentum generated by the record-breaking year for women's sports in 2019.

Of course, this report was published before Covid-19 attacked the planet but the principles remained the same and should apply now that things have returned to normal.

While this would all be wonderful for women's sport, beware the wolf lurking in sheep's clothing. Do you really think they want to grow women's sport to help women in sport? Maybe some of them do and are genuinely well-intentioned but remember, sports administrators are politicians, they are to be treated with suspicion.

The growth of women's sport equals business growth equals more money. Where is that money going to go? Think on that if you are hoping to become a serious investigative reporter.

Another area that affected female athletes, especially teenage girls, was the disgusting matter of sexual abuse. USA Gymnastics (USAG) had been under intense pressure for its handling of the Larry Nassar affair. If you are not familiar with the story, Nassar was convicted after being found guilty of sexually abusing several female youth gymnasts (including future Olympic gold medallists) while he was the USAG national team doctor.

You can go and read more about this vile individual but suffice to say, there are hundreds of Larry Nassars out there. You can create a niche for yourself by being the sports reporter that exposes these horrible human beings, and while it is true that young girls were the most vulnerable, there are young boys out there who are also being abused by these nefarious individuals. Who said that sports journalism was not serious?

An area that is often difficult to comprehend for non-U.S. sports fans is the college sports scene. Usually in Europe and other parts of the world, after completing school, an aspiring young player will immediately try to become a professional athlete. Often, the player has already been part of a club system and a big contract with a Premier League club or even Champions League club cannot be too far away.

That is not quite how it works Stateside where college sport is the virtually exclusive pathway to the professional leagues. It must be odd for someone not from the United States watching a televised NFL game for the first time and noticing the players introducing themselves before kick-off.

What is striking is how each player would provide their name as well as the college from which they graduated, for example "Tua Tagovailoa, University of Alabama". This is unthinkable elsewhere. As a South African, the first time I watched an NFL game and witnessed this, I wondered to myself why on Earth would anyone care what school, college or university a player attended.

In fairness that might be because I did not attend the most prestigious school and found references to elite high schools by my peers and colleagues rather irritating and even elitist.

In October 2019, the National Collegiate Athletic Association (NCAA) announced plans to eventually allow college athletes to earn compensation for the use of their name, image, or likeness. The NCAA's announcement came on the heels of California's Fair Pay to Play Act, signed in September 2019 that would allow college players to strike endorsement deals and hire agents.

College sport was such a massive deal in the United States that student athletes would earn compensation on things like name and image rights, and likeness-or put another way, there could be a video game with them featuring as a character. I bet if you are not from the USA, the thought that a student could be featured in a sports video game is virtually unfathomable.

In many ways, it had already happened. Ed O'Bannon challenged the usage of his likeness in a college basketball video game, and in 2013, EA Sports was forced to discontinue its successful college football video game franchise. Based on recent developments, is there a chance that college sports video games would re-emerge, using the likenesses of actual athletes?

I think there is no doubt and investigative reporters will want to keep an eye on the licences, fees, agents and leagues. Who knows who or what may be lurking?

With the early rollout of 5G, there were more digital possibilities in sport than ever before. Keep an eye out for Virtual Reality, Augmented Reality and Artificial Intelligence; they are already here but set for significant expansion. Imagine fans arriving at stadiums wearing headsets. The fans at home could be wearing the headsets in order to enjoy the same stadium experience.

It is very exciting but also teams, leagues and federations would no doubt be offering tenders to VR, AR and AI providers. Who will they be? Where will the money really be going? By now, you should have sniffed an opportunity for some investigation, after all, these developments raise a host of questions—and potential opportunities; for athletes, sponsors, and advertisers alike. Not to mention the villains.

Hitherto, this chapter has focused mostly on Europe and North America but I want to spend some time discussing the Asian market, starting with India.

When one thinks of India in sporting terms, usually the country's famous national cricket team springs to mind. Thoughts turn to greats like Sunil Gavaskar, Sachin Tendulkar and Virat Kohli. India have won the Cricket World Cup twice (1983 and 2011), as well as the World Twenty20 (2007) and two Champions Trophy titles (2002, 2013) among other achievements.

More on cricket later but first let us look at football's Indian Super League (ISL), a competition that had an impressive cumulative TV viewership of 429 million in its inaugural season in 2014 and viewership that grew 26% y/y in the 2015 season.

Average attendance at an ISL game was 24,357 in its first season – only below Germany's Bundesliga, Spain's La Liga and the English Premier League, would you believe?

Elsewhere, the first season of Pro Kabaddi League (PKL) in 2014 was watched by 435 million people, and its viewership increased 20% y/y in its second season and 35% y/y in its third season.

While cricket dominates the sports market in India, the country had clearly embraced other sports with much zeal and enthusiasm. During the period 2013–15, eight major league-based sports tournaments were launched in India.

They were admittedly met with varying degrees of success, and even failure but what should be of more interest to you as a sports reporter is that the sports sector in India is governed by both the central and state governments, meaning it is often hampered by bureaucracy and politics.

In other words, the ideal environment for all kinds of villainy to take place. Issues around irregular activities have already been reported in the past.

Because there are federations at several government or state tiers, it often brings about conflict so for example, the Indian Hockey Federation (IHF) and Hockey India (HI) were involved in a seven-year long battle for recognition that only ended in September 2015 when the Court of Arbitration for Sport (CAS) announced its verdict that allowed HI to retain its status as hockey's national body in India.

Investigative sports reporter Heaven, and just for some added flavour, many sports federations in India were not headed by sports persons but often by people involved in politics as well. In 2015, more than one-half of the recognised federations had politicians at the helm.

I promised some cricket numbers. The 2015 ICC Cricket World Cup was watched by a cumulative 635 million Indians until India lost the semi-final match against Australia. In 2016, this was followed by the ICC World Twenty20, which witnessed a cumulative viewership of 730 million.

Moreover, the Indian Premier League's (IPL) 2016 season garnered 347 million viewers, a 22% growth on the previous season. Unsurprisingly, as a result of the IPL's massive returns, the incumbent official broadcaster Sony Pictures Networks (SPN) India was keen on continuing its association with the mega league after its initial contract expired in 2017.

In 2015, the overall sports sponsorship market in India grew approximately 12.5% to approximately $7 billion. On-air sponsorship had consistently accounted for the bulk (52% in 2015) of total sports advertising in India. It grew 6.7 per cent in 2015, and the rising popularity of several league-based tournaments, such as the ISL, PKL and Hockey India League (HIL) drove the results.

Also, on ground sponsorship witnessed a stark rise of approximately 30% y/y in 2015; driven by football and kabaddi, wherein on ground sponsorship rose by 91.6% and 300% respectively.

India is the second-largest market for broadcast media after China, with 675 million people having access to TV in India (as of August 2016). India is also currently the second-largest market globally by the number of internet subscribers again, only behind China.

More than 50% of an IPL team's revenue typically comes from the share of the broadcasting fees and central sponsorship income from the BCCI.

The Indian sports broadcasting space comprises three major players: Star India, SPN and ZEE Entertainment. Star India has a portfolio of almost all the major sports properties, except for the IPL, which was under SPN's kitty. In August 2016, ZEE announced its intent to sell its Ten Sports portfolio to SPN for approximately $3 billion-effectively making the market a duopoly, as other broadcasters such as Neo Sports had a very small share of the market.

You may very well be reading this book after some of these events have already taken place. Do not be discouraged. Broadcast and sponsorship deals work in cycles. There is always a contract that is expiring or coming up for renegotiation.

If your dream is to become an investigative sports reporter, find out when these expiry dates are, draw up a list, identify the ones that most interest you and start working on your next story.

The Indian market information came courtesy of a sports business report by KPMG India.37

Another region within Asia that has very successfully used sport to promote itself, is the Middle East. The United Arab Emirates (UAE) and Qatar have led the way with several high-profile annual sports events but Saudi Arabia has also realised just how powerful sport can be to paint a country in a positive light.

---

[37] Gillett, A.G. (2017). The business of sports agents. Business History, 61(2), pp.374–375.

Many people often incorrectly refer to Dubai as a country. Dubai is a city in the UAE. Abu Dhabi is the capital city of the UAE and please do not confuse Doha, Qatar's capital with Dubai.

At the time of writing, Doha is my home and it astonishes me how many people interchange, or confuse, Dubai and Doha. They are not even in the same country. Ordinary citizens are barely forgiven for such errors but for reporters, it is an inexcusable error. Know your geography.

Sport has an economic footprint of more than $1.7 billion a year in Dubai alone. These figures reflected the success of a carefully developed sports industry, with Dubai investing in sustainable facilities that attract elite sports events and contributed to the sports participation agenda of the UAE.

This strategy is prevalent in a number of sports such as golf, tennis and rugby along with the more recent example of cycling. Sport accounts for approximately 0.8% of Dubai's GDP. Sponsorship is a well-developed market, with globally recognised brands from Dubai and overseas sponsoring events.

Total value is estimated at approximately $100 million, and the sport industry in Dubai is estimated to employ around 14,500 people, or 0.6% of the city's total workforce.[38]

Obviously, some sports enjoy bigger exposure and revenue than others, but why should they have all the fun? Table tennis was keen to take its place at the top table, or at the very least, get its slice of the pie. The International Table Tennis Federation (ITTF) released a report in 2018[39] documenting its growth strategy. It went to great lengths to promote itself, as it should do, of course.

The ITTF claimed it was the first and only international sports federation to achieve 226 national associations. That would make it bigger than the United Nations, but then you have to start questioning the legitimacy and autonomy of places like American Samoa, Puerto Rico and Chinese Taipei-or is it Taiwan?

Nevertheless, the ITTF claimed to have more than 30 million competitive players worldwide and had TV viewership of 355 million for its 2017 World Championships.

---

[38] Deloitte United Kingdom. (n.d.). Falcon and Associates/Dubai Sports Council-Economic Impact of Sport in Dubai. [online] Available at: https://www2.deloitte.com/uk/en/pages/sports-business-group/articles/economic-impact-of-sport-in-dubai.html [Accessed 22 May 2020].

[39] ITTF Strategic Plan. (2018). [online] Available at: https://www.ittf.com/wp-content/uploads/2018/08/ITTF-Strategic-Plan-en.pdf.

The ITTF hoped to increase its sponsorship and broadcast revenue by 100% by 2024 and significantly, increase broadcast reach by 50% by 2024.

It would be wonderful to see table tennis establish itself as a mainstream sport. It is fun to watch and action-packed, but by now you must also know that with this kind of aggressive growth and potential revenue intake, there is bound to be a bad guy lurking. Who would be the investigative sports reporter to uncover the murkiness? It could be you.

Rugby union is in a perennial struggle against rugby league just to be seen as the number one rugby code. Given the success of union and the growth of its global market and world cup, certainly for now it is safe to say it is winning the battle, but will it win the war?

According to Matthew T. Brown40, the global rugby union community comprised 9.6 million players and 338 million fans affiliated via 127 national member unions in six regions and driven by the commercial success of the Rugby World Cup, World Rugby was planning to invest £620 million at all levels of the game between 2020 and 2023*, eclipsing the previous four-year cycle by 28%, to ensure strong and sustainable growth.

During the writing of this book, Argentina's former captain turned administrator, Agustin Pichot lost his bid to become the chairman of World Rugby. The sport's governing body opted to hand Sir Bill Beaumont, a former England captain, a second term.

Many from the southern hemisphere, and other developing nations, saw this as a slap in the face and predicted more of the same, instead of much needed change that Pichot claimed he would be able to deliver. Might this be the gap rugby league needs?

That code's Super League in England, already includes a French club and now a Canadian club, the Toronto Wolfpack, who were so ambitious they lured All Blacks star, Sonny Bill Williams from union to join their fledgling organisation as the Super League's highest ever paid player.[41]

---

[40] Anon, (n.d.). [online] Available at:
http://www.measure4you.de/images/AnalysisOfOnlineMarketingInTheSportsIndustry.pdf.

[41] Press, A.A. (2019). 'Rugby's LeBron James': Toronto confirm Sonny Bill Williams signing. [online]
The Guardian. Available at: https://www.theguardian.com/sport/2019/nov/08/rugbys-lebron-james-toronto-confirm-sonny-bill-williams-signing [Accessed 26 May 2020].

Earlier in the chapter, we discussed ANOC and ASOIF. If it is already vague, let me refresh your memory. ANOC is the Association of National Olympic Committees, while ASOIF is the Association of Summer Olympic International Federations (ASOIF). The latter released their own report in 2019 entitled *Future of Global Sport*.[42]

Of course, you want to treat the ASOIF with the suspicion they deserve. After all, there was already an IOC, then curiously there was also an ANOC, and then on top of that, an ASOIF too. Nevertheless, let us cast our cynicism aside and look at what they have to say first.

The ASOIF report looked at the history of sport ruling bodies before discussing its commercial development, chiefly through live television. It was an interesting read and I would recommend you take it in, even if just for enrichment purposes.

Things became very interesting around the time of the 1992 Olympic Games in Barcelona. This was the first time the IOC shared out revenues to international federations (IF). The total doled out to the IFs totalled $1.5 million. Even in those days that was not overly significant but it laid a very notable foundation.

By mid-2017, it had been able to pay out a total of over $540 million in revenue shares to the 28 sports on the Olympic Games programme from the Rio 2016 Games alone.

It was very interesting that the ASOIF recognised that the goose that laid the golden egg may at some point run dry. Cities like Hamburg, Rome and Budapest withdrew from bidding to host the 2024 Olympics, citing costs. Hamburg held a referendum to determine its stance. How is that for democracy in action?

In the end, Paris won the right to host the Games and whether the IOC panicked or not, it awarded Los Angeles, the only other city left in the race, the 2028 Olympics. While many Parisians and Angelenos were excited about hosting the global sporting showpiece, not everyone felt the same way.

I would encourage you to take a look at the Nolympics LA movement. This is a group quite obviously opposed to their city hosting the Games. They claim that the Olympics destroy communities and kill cities. They may very well have a point and they are likely to grant you an interview at any time, especially if you

---

[42] Future Of Global Sport Association Of Summer Olympic International Federations. (2019). [Online] Available At:
Https://Www.Asoif.Com/Sites/Default/Files/Download/Future_Of_Global_Sport.Pdf.

have caught wind of irregularities at the IOC, but beware of allying yourself with organisations like Nolympics.

It would be akin to siding with Greenpeace if you were an environmental journalist. Sometimes, there can be a fine line between being a journalist and an activist.

It was not just the summer Olympic Games that had challenges. Perhaps the Winter Games had an even bigger headache. Not only does it also face the same difficulties in terms of costs, but these were compounded by the environmental challenges presented by winter sports.

The ASOIF report references an article in The Economist pointing out that greenhouse gas emissions were more pronounced in the Alps than the average, where a rise of two degrees Celsius was common.

In addition, the Organisation for Economic Co-operation and Development, or OECD as you have likely heard them referred to as, projected back in 2006 that 40% of 666 alpine ski resorts would no longer be able to operate a 100-day ski season if temperatures rose a further two degrees Celsius and 70% could disappear if the rise were to be four degrees Celsius.

In terms of hosting winter sports, another study concluded that only 13 of the 21 former hosts looked certain to be able to host winter sports in 2050. While some sports had moved their events from the traditional centres of Europe and North America to the Middle East, Far East and other exotic locations, in a bid to save costs, increase revenues and expand their global audience, winter sports, and indeed the Winter Olympic Games, may not have as many options available. It is unlikely to snow in Doha anytime soon.

Sport is clearly full of gangsters and villains who are keen to grab power in federations in a bid to line their own pockets. Yes, that is a true statement, but in spite of a rather cynical theme in this chapter, not all administrators are nefarious. You would do well to remember that many of them truly love the sport or clubs they serve and want what is best.

The reality is that some will do a great job, and others will do a bad job, because they are just simply out of their depth, while others are there to take advantage of the commercial benefits. As a journalist, you would want to be mindful of that.

Similarly, not all athletes are going to compete fairly. The lure of a world cup trophy or Olympic gold medal could become so overwhelming that athletes resort to cheating, or in the case of Mohammad Amir and Hansie Cronje, they deliberately play badly in exchange for material rewards.

We have also established there are vast amounts of money involved in sport and outside of the administrators and athletes, it would be worth your while to keep an eye on the sponsors, media rights holders and agents that tend to be outside of the public's eye but very strong role players.

Remember a bribe could secure media rights, or sponsorship, just as easily as it could guarantee a vote in the next World Cup bid selection meeting.

These are very strong reasons for becoming a sports journalist and those reasons are certainly worthy of being used in any conversation in which you feel you need to justify your choice to a peer who deemed sport to be second-tier. That said there is still a lot of romance in sport.

If you are like me, you have been following sport since the age of eight and made sure over the years to watch the games (including the highlights and magazine programmes), listened to the radio interviews, bought all the magazines and tournament brochures you could get your hands on, and naturally attended as many games as you possibly could.

It is natural that as a lover of sport, and now keen to enter journalism, that it is your love of sport rather than investigation that got you here. That is okay. You do not have to feel guilty about that but just remember to separate the fan from the reporter when you are working.

I thought I would include some lighter reasons for why sport is important, and why it needs journalism, to conclude the chapter since there was some very serious stuff hitherto.

In *The Political Economy of Television Sports Rights*[43], the authors discussed the role sport played as a unifying factor. They referenced how rugby was famously used by South Africa's first democratically-elected president Nelson Mandela to help bring black and white members of the population together during the 1995 Rugby World Cup.

The achievement by Mandela and the Springboks became the subject of a best-selling book, *Playing The Enemy*, and Hollywood blockbuster film *Invictus*. Many other sports events and achievements had become the subject of books and films too.

---

[43] Evens, T., Petros Iosifidis and Smith, P. (2013). The political economy of television sports rights. Basingstoke, Palgrave Macmillan

The authors also pointed out that all the 1995 Rugby World Cup matches were shown on SABC, the country's national terrestrial broadcaster. We spoke about television rights earlier in the chapter. There is an important role to play for terrestrial channels because more people have access to it than subscription services.

In Chapter 11, the authors also highlight how sport had been used by broadcasters to contribute towards the wider objectives of nation-building, reconciliation, democratisation and cultural diversity but these objectives had taken place against the backdrop of an increasingly marketised broadcasting system.

In many countries, free-to-air television coverage of sports events and competitions, most notably by public service broadcasters and terrestrial commercial networks, had facilitated shared viewing experiences, which have fostered a sense of national identity and cultural citizenship.

Sport most certainly brought people together when my country South Africa won the Rugby WorldCup in 2019 (as they did in 1995 and 2007). The country's people celebrated as one. In that moment, the citizens forgot their daily problems and cheered on its rugby heroes. As far as I am aware, no general election could do that.

Even the famous 1994 election, which was my country's first democratic election and celebrated globally, saw approximately 38% of the voters choose a party other than Nelson Mandela's African National Congress. Yes, the election was free and fair, it was peaceful, and Mandela became a national hero even to those who did not vote for his party, but I think we could safely speculate that the national rugby team had more fans than the governing party.

Similarly, who do you think had more fans in 2014: Germany's FIFA World Cup-winning team or the country's then-chancellor Angela Merkel? With respect to Mrs Merkel, I doubt it was even a contest.

It is also worth singling out the point made by Boardman and Hargreaves-Heap[44] that "people not only like to watch major sports events, they also like to talk about them, and the conversational value of an event depends in part on the number of people who also watch it".

Sure, people talk religion and politics, despite the commonly held wisdom to avoid those two topics, but they love discussing sport too. How many people

---

[44] Boardman, A.E. and Hargreaves-Heap, S.P. (1999). Journal of Cultural Economics, 23(3), pp.165– 179.

have you heard over the years discuss a goal that should have been ruled out because a player was offside?

Or the common complaints now over the Video Assistant Referee (VAR) that has not managed to eradicate refereeing errors despite its sales pitch? I wonder how many people in Italy and South Korea, or the world for that matter, were talking about Ahn Jung-hwan's winning goal in extra time at the 2002 World Cup.

Chapter 14 in *Sport, Public Broadcasting, And Cultural Citizenship: Signal Lost?* [45] by Muhammed Musa, entitled *The Political Economy of Football Viewership in Africa*[46], cites Sullivan's work that suggested that the outcome of a sporting contest brought about a particular set of emotions (negative or positive depending on the outcome) and this was further enhanced by the narrative provided by the television commentators.

From a psychological perspective, this is similar to the way politicians and other local or national representatives exploit people's interviews in televised interviews.[47]

Back to the topic of terrestrial television. Australia has the most comprehensive set of laws and regulations designed to prevent the migration of sporting events from free-to-air television to pay-TV. The appropriate government minister has the authority to "specify an event, or events, that in the opinion of the minister, must be available free to the general public".[48]

Thus, iconic events such as horse racing's Melbourne Cup, the National Rugby League and Australian Football League finals must be televised on free-to-air broadcasters.

---

[45] Scherer, J. and Sam, M.P., 2012. Public Broadcasting, Sport and Cultural Citizenship: Sky's the Limit in New Zealand. Media Culture & Society. 34(10), pp.101-111

[46] Musa, M., 2014. Sport, Public Broadcasting, and Cultural Citizenship: Signal Lost? Location: ROUTLEDGE.

[47] Sullivan, G., 2009. Germany, Television and the 2006 World Cup: National Narrative of Pride and Party Patriotism. In: E. Castello, A. Dhoest, and H. O'Donnell, eds., The Nation on Screen, Discourses of the National in Global Television. Cambridge: Cambridge Scholars Press.

[48] Evens, T., Petros Iosifidis and Smith, P. (2013). The political economy of television sports rights. Basingstoke, Palgrave Macmillan.

Sport is so important that politicians have passed laws making it mandatory for certain events to be broadcast on terrestrial television. Those sports have been designated as culturally significant or key to the national psyche in some cases. This should warm your heart. You can justify your chosen path with confidence and enthusiasm, and maybe even convert one or two of your peers to join the pool of sports journalists.

It would be worth your while to look at the various study options that are open to you. Do not worry if you are reading this as a fourth-year honours, or fifth-year masters student, I am not about to set you on a 180-degree course correction. You have not wasted any time or effort, I can promise you. Your efforts are still very much on course to be rewarded.

Chapter Three
Taking Sides

Journalists are expected to be objective. The only real exception to this would be the opinion journalists so prevalent on U.S. network news channels. Newspaper or online columnists also sometimes fall under this category. So yes, there is some room for manoeuvring, but you do not ever want to come across as biased or even worse, a fan.

Your audience can detect your biases and will not hold back in their criticism. A simple glance at the comments section of just about any website, or social media post, will bear testament to that. They can be very cruel with their comments.

You will have to have a thick skin. You might even find that you have written a 5000-word feature and someone is having a go at you for one phrase in that piece. Get used to it.

In this chapter, we shall look at the realities facing a reporter covering a local team. There are certain expectations from the readers but also from your editors. Remember that local media tends to "support" the home team, but you have to draw the line somewhere.

One reporter who did not wish to be interviewed for this book told me that he did not have to draw a line since he was not even from the same town as the team he covered and did not support them anyway. That was an advantage I had when I moved from Cape Town, where I grew up, to Johannesburg and began covering Joburg and Pretoria-based teams. It made no difference to me if those sides were winning or losing.

You will hear from two reporters in this chapter; one who grew up supporting English Premier League team Newcastle United, and one who grew up in New York City before moving with his family to Miami, where he has been ever since and has covered the Miami Dolphins in the National Football League.

Bear in mind that reporters and columnists will often report things that do not sit well with some players, coaches or administrators who tend to become grumpy when their team is not doing well. It would be your task to report that they were performing badly.

They could moan and groan all they like but we are not in the pre-1735 era anymore. This was when freedom of the press was first advanced in a major manner. In a landmark case, John Peter Zenger, a New York City newspaper publisher, was acquitted of libel on the defence that his political criticism was based on fact.

That was 41 years before the United States even became the United States. Press freedom in the States was then further secured by the First Amendment to the U.S. Constitution in 1791. In most western countries, this kind of guarantee is enjoyed by the press but no matter what country you hail from, make sure you know the relevant laws. Most of the time if it is true, you can report it because you can argue that it was in the interest of the public.

In my view, the concept of objectivity is not absolute. For example, the *Miami Herald* would always be in the Dolphins' corner. Similarly, *The Chronicle* are cheering for Newcastle United. Remember those two publications are selling a product to people who support those teams and want to read about them.

That means that the headlines will read "Dolphins Lose" or "Newcastle Beaten" rather than the other team winning. In and of itself that is okay as long as the journalists are capable of being critical of their local teams when they are not doing well; whether that be on the field in terms of results or bad behaviour at board level.

Similarly, from a political perspective media houses have always leaned liberal or conservative, capitalist or socialist and so on. Up to a certain point, it is acceptable. Many newspapers openly endorse political parties or candidates. Is that being objective?

There was stiff competition in New York City in the 19th century between Joseph Pulitzer, who owned the *World* from 1883, and William Randolph Hearst, who owned the *Journal* around 1895. Their fierce rivalry led to excesses of lurid and sensationalised news, called yellow journalism, and reactions against it in the late 1890s. I think we can safely refer to that as 19th century click bait. And you thought that was a 21st century phenomenon!

A dissatisfaction among younger readers with established papers led to the emergence in the second half of the 20th century of a diverse "underground", or alternative press. The alternative press was forthright in seeking fresh approaches.

Various special-interest groups including ethnic, religious and trade interests, were also served by papers edited specifically for them.[49] Would you call that objective journalism or catering to a target market?

Mehdi Hasan has a particularly confrontational style of interviewing. You can look up his *Head To Head* and *Up Front* programmes on Al Jazeera to get an idea. A lot of it can be found on YouTube. While he does come across as ready for battle, he is equally excellently prepared. Does he have an agenda? I think he does and again, that is not necessarily a negative thing.

He has been described as abrasive and pugilistic, with a zeal for Twitter confrontations that is often beneath him. He sees these "outsider" qualities as strengths that enable him to transcend the pitfalls of a U.S. news media paralysed by an old-fashioned courteousness towards those in political office.

As he said, "The British press, the British media, for all its flaws, does not have this culture of deference when it comes to interviewing a person in power. I am amazed that the press stands up when the president enters the room. They don't do that for Boris Johnson".[50]

Hasan is a practicing Muslim. Have his religious beliefs influenced his reporting? As a man of faith myself, I find it hard to imagine, at the very least, that his questions have not been influenced by the way he sees the world. I would argue that is inevitable. That is not necessarily a bad thing as long as the right questions are being asked, which I think Hasan does.

He is also "unabashedly left wing". That is fine but it is important to emphasise that the left wing, liberal viewpoint is not necessarily the right one and certainly not the only one. It is merely an opinion or a frame of reference. I hope that if Hasan reads this, he will not feel compelled to punch me in the nose!

Regarding agenda setting, there are lessons to be taken from Chapter 11 of *The Handbook of Journalism Studies*. The process of the mass media presenting

[49] newspaper | History & Facts. (2019). In: Encyclopædia Britannica. [online] Available at: https://www.britannica.com/topic/newspaper.

[50] The Guardian. (2020). Mehdi Hasan: 'Most people ask the question and move on. I don't.' [online] Available at: https://www.theguardian.com/tv-and-radio/2020/mar/27/mehdi-hasan-interview [Accessed 27 May 2020].

certain issues frequently and prominently result in how large segments of the public come to perceive those issues as more important than others. Simply put, the more coverage an issue receives, the more important it is to people. (p.147) [51]

Weaver found that increased concern over the federal budget deficit was linked to increased knowledge of the possible causes and solutions of this problem, which resulted in stronger and more polarised opinions about it, and more likelihood of engaging in some form of political behaviour.[52]

While this is not sport-related, it does highlight how what is put at the forefront of news media content, will inevitably gain the status of being more important and you can appreciate the power held in the proverbial pen of journalists.

Boardman and Hargreaves-Heap wrote that "people not only like to watch major sports events, they also like to talk about them, and the conversational value of an event depends in part on the number of people who also watch it".

This amounted to a gatekeeping of information as alluded to by Shoemaker, Vos and Reese: Journalists are bombarded with information from the Internet, newspapers, television and radio news, news magazines, and their sources. Their job of selecting and shaping the small amount of information that becomes news would be impossible without gatekeeping. It is the process of selecting, writing, editing, positioning, scheduling, repeating and otherwise massaging information to become news.

From that, you can also see that it is virtually impossible for a reporter or columnist to cover every aspect of a story and inevitably, they must decide what elements are more important and newsworthy.

Now that you have a decent background on what might shape the views of a reporter or columnist, consciously or subconsciously, let me introduce you to the two journalists who kindly agreed to be interviewed for this chapter.

---

[51] Coleman, R., McCombs, M., Shaw, D. and Weaver, D., 2009. *The Handbook of Journalism Studies* [e-book] New York: Routledge. Available through: Edinburgh Napier University Library website <https://ebookcentral.proquest.com/lib/napier/reader.action?docID=401841&query=> [Accessed 19 September 2018].

[52] Weaver, D. (1991). Issue salience and public opinion: Are there consequences of agenda-setting?
International Journal of Public Opinion, 3, pp.53– 68

Armando Salguero is a senior NFL writer at *Outkick*. When he kindly agreed to be interviewed for this book, he was a *Miami Herald* sports columnist covering the Miami Dolphins. Chris Waugh is the Newcastle United correspondent for *The Athletic*.

He spoke to me during the pandemic in 2020 some 18 months before English billionaire Mike Ashley sold the club he covers to a Saudi-Arabian-led consortium. I asked both men if they were fans of the teams they cover before taking up positions as local reporters.

Salguero was not, although he was an NFL fan. He moved with his parents to Miami in the summer of 1972, which just happened to be a great time to be a Dolphins supporter as he explained, 'So, we're new in Miami and all I hear about in the fall of 1972 is the Miami Dolphins in South Florida. Miami Dolphins this, Miami Dolphins that.

'It just so happens that 1972 was the year that the Miami Dolphins were undefeated and as a 10-year-old who had just come from New York, I guess it struck a rebellious chord in me. At that time, the team that was often on the other channel around the same time on a Sunday afternoon was the Washington Redskins.

'A lot of their games were broadcast down here and low and behold, come the Super Bowl, it was the Dolphins playing the Redskins for the Championship and so, while I wasn't rooting for the Redskins at that point, I couldn't just be "part of the gang" but obviously the Dolphins were in my backyard so I followed them but, was I a fan of the Dolphins? I guess 10-year-old Armando would say no.'

Waugh has a very different story. He grew up in Newcastle and his father would take him to games. He confessed to having been a huge fan with a season ticket, 'The first time I got it was for my 11th birthday and the first ever game I went to was Rob Lee's testimonial.

'My dad and I would sit in the Gallowgate End for years and even when I was away at university, my dad kept the season ticket going and if I wasn't here, my brother would go or my sister would go but most of the time, I would try and come back when I could.

'As I got older, I didn't go to every single away game but I would go to one in three when I could and when I lived down in London, even when I could, I would go to games. I was, and I suppose I still am a supporter.'

Waugh believed his history as a boyhood fan of the local side had been beneficial as a lot of research on the history of the club was not necessary as he already had it stored in his memory.

Understandably, working as a local reporter covering the team he grew up supporting had its own challenges in terms of remaining objective. Waugh was quite philosophical about it, 'I don't think there's a right or wrong way to do it, but some people are quite overt about the fact that they're a fan.'

I can understand why but I've always tried to be as objective as I can even when I was working at *The Chronicle* where whatever I was writing had a Newcastle United bias or slant. If you were to write a match report for Newcastle-Liverpool, and I focused on Liverpool for a local newspaper on Tyneside, then it doesn't make any sense, so there's always that bias to a degree.

My personal view is that I can better inform people having the view that I have as a supporter and having that history, but also to try and take a step back and be as objective as possible and so I found it difficult to begin with and to a certain extent, certainly for a period, managed to almost entirely disengage from being a fan and I managed to properly step away and that was hard because obviously I've grown up my whole life following Newcastle United and that's been such a big part of my life and it remained a big part of my life but in a different way.

I was no longer a fan. I was someone covering the club and I felt I needed to do that to begin with just to give myself that distance and over time I've been able to find more of a happy medium. I'm still not overt about the fact that I'm a Newcastle United fan even though I think it comes across quite clearly because of my accent and my knowledge of the team maybe.

'I don't refer to Newcastle United as "we" necessarily and I do think that's important for the way I feel I can best cover the club. Obviously, I do have biases and I can't pretend that I'm completely objective because I don't think any journalist covering anything can be completely objective.'

Waugh's mention of stepping away entirely and going the other way is a warning. It could happen that in your determination to cover your favourite local team objectively, you become overly critical and negative. While it is good to try your best to cover your childhood team as objectively as possible, be careful not to become so "blinded by neutrality" that you start seeing things that are not there.

Salguero had a great solution to this in that he praised the Dolphins when they were doing well, but when they were not doing well, he called himself their "worst nightmare". He found it easier to hide any biases since he was not actually a boyhood Dolphins fan, even though he does root for them in his own way, 'I want the Dolphins to do well.

'I don't hide that fact and why do I want the Dolphins to do well? Well, because that means I do well! It is to my benefit if I am covering a team that has more recognition, more prominence, more consequence and the way you get that in sports is with success.

'Unfortunately for the Dolphins, they did a lot of that in the 20th century, but not nearly as much in the 21st century. Since 2000, they were under.500 as a franchise, so what my job has become a lot of, is detailing failure, and it's not fun and folks aren't happy to do it, or help you do it, but it happened so what are you gonna do? And the fans obviously understand that; fans being in my mind equated to readers and people who take in the information that I put out.'

Salguero references the fans who are his readership or his audience. There are editors who believe that journalists must cater specifically to their audience. Put another way, writers must give the readers what they want. That can be challenging.

I asked both men how they balanced being objective with supplying their audience with what they want and they both provided truly journalistic answers.

Salguero believes that if you had that debate in your mind, the scales will always be tipped in favour of the wrong argument, 'I give my audience what they want but here's the thing, last year (2019) the Miami Dolphins, in their first game, lost the game 59-10.

'Does my audience want to know what went right? Or do they want to know what went wrong and why? Because that's what I would want to know. The idea of feeding your audience what they want isn't necessarily sugar-coating stuff and lying to them. I think people want the truth.

'These people are adults. They don't want to be lied to. They don't want to be pampered. They don't have diapers that I have to change when things go bad because they've soiled themselves. What has happened is something went wrong. Let me explain it to you.

'Let the Dolphins or whomever I cover give you their side of it and then obviously you have eyes, you saw what happened. Let's get a reasoning for this. It's not about giving you a shoulder to cry on. That's not what I do. What I do is, here, this is what happened, and this is why, and if you wanna know the truth then you're gonna take this in.

'I'm gonna tell 'em the truth and if that upsets them, okay. If that fulfils them, okay. But I'm gonna be true to myself and tell them what is honest and tell them what is true. When things are good, I'm gonna tell 'em things are really good.

'When things are bad, I'm gonna tell 'em things are bad and I think that as a brand, a journalist who decides to do that, rather than taking an advocacy position is way better off because truth is a great shield and a great sword. Advocacy is neither.'

Waugh compared the Rafael Benitez and Steve McClaren eras as Newcastle United coaches as an example where he thought local reporters were thinking more about spoon feeding the audience, 'There was a period when Rafa Benitez first came to Newcastle that we would mirror some of the things the fans did.

'So, we would refer to him as "Rafa" and after a little bit of time, I realised that I was doing the same and I felt that actually that was making it too personable. I think there needs to be that distance. The previous manager, Steve McClaren was never referred to as "Steve" most of the time.

'Probably now and again you might, but generally you'd refer to him as "McClaren" so I've tried ever since to refer to them as "Benitez" or "Bruce" (as in Steve, the man who succeeded Benitez).'

One of the key components to being a local reporter is to build relationships and trust with the coach, players, administrators and often other staff too like the media liaison, for example. The relationships could be dynamic, depending on the personalities being dealt with and the situation could be equally dynamic given the high turnaround of head coaches in many sports leagues.

Salguero called his relationship with the role players at the Dolphins respectful, 'I am not there to mock them. I'm not there to make them look bad, neither am I there to crown them, or lie to you and tell you things are better than what they are. I think that if your brand is the truth, you're gonna be all right.

'These people are adults, and they're very smart, and they're very good at what they do. They know more than I do when things are going wrong. Also, they know more than I do when things are going right. So, I rely on what they know but also what the resulting product is, and I understand that.

'For example, the Dolphins' last four or five head coaches have had great first seasons in that they had success and then after that it's gone downhill. Well, during those great first seasons there's a lot of applause going on, but they understand that when things go downhill, there's no longer a lot of applause, there's a lot of "thumbs down" going on and I think they're adult enough to know it because they know it's not going in the right direction and they're doing everything they can to fix it.'

Waugh shared how in some cases at Newcastle United, it had been impossible to build relationships with some people, and in other instances impossible to even access people, like the then-club owner Mike Ashley for example, 'With the coaches in general, certainly with Benitez, there was a bit more distance.

'Certainly, when you were in a press conference with him, he was always great but he's not someone who you can necessarily just pick the phone up to and just do it in that sort of way. Steve Bruce is slightly different. I don't really have the kind of relationship that some of the reporters do who worked with him at Sunderland and other clubs like Hull.

'They can ring him on a daily basis and speak to him. I don't necessarily have that. I can message him and speak to him but he is a lot more approachable in that sense and there isn't a bad relationship. Steve Bruce has fallen out with other local journalists but in general dealing with the managers has been fine.

'Players-wise, whenever we get to speak to them on the rare occasions we do, they tend to be good. Some of them are a lot more receptive to stopping and talking, particularly after games. There are others who don't like to speak. Jonjo Shelvey doesn't really like to speak.

'There was a weird incident where it was Newcastle's first season back in the Premier League and they were playing Brighton away. It was not long after Shelvey had been sent off against Spurs and the irony is that I wasn't there for that game. I was actually on holiday, so I did not give any coverage to that game.

'When I asked Shelvey to stop at the mixed zone at Brighton, I think I got the anger in him from everyone else's coverage so he was like, "Oh, you wanna talk now after everything you've written", and I thought, *Well actually it wasn't me and Jonjo Shelvey hasn't really wanted to speak to me ever since so that's been a bit difficult.*

'In terms of the administrators, Mike Ashley is just impossible to get to. He doesn't speak and trying to get to him is unfortunately just impossible. As for (managing director) Lee Charnley, I don't have the kind of relationship where I can just call him. I do have his number, but I don't have that sort of relationship.

'I have been in to see him before and I've had briefings from him and whenever I've spoken to him, I've found him to be someone pretty decent to deal with. I think he is honest. I think he doesn't sugar-coat things. He does say things honestly, buthe doesn't like to speak too often.

'He doesn't like to explain too much and whenever, on the rare occasions when I have met him, it's always been on his terms and after a while I sort of said I don't want to continue doing this because it was just a case of if we speak on this for now, in time we will build up a relationship whereby nothing is off limits and I just said to myself as an independent journalist that can't be the way this will keep going on.

'I'm not here to just peddle whatever you want to say. I'm here to serve a purpose which is to connect with the fans. So, it was never a negative relationship necessarily, but it wasn't a close one or one where it got on to the sort of terms where it would have been healthier.'

The reality was that these role players needed to understand that at the end of the day, reporters were there to do a job. Salguero and Waugh both felt that generally the Dolphins and Newcastle had been mostly professional in that sense.

While they were mostly professionally, they are still human and open to having emotional reactions or trying to push their own agendas. 'Steve Bruce has been a bit perturbed by some of the coverage in general and has taken some of it to heart and I can understand why.

'Benitez was very good at directing the narrative in the way that he wanted it to go, so I don't think he ever really had that issue where it reached the point where he wouldn't have been happy with it being out there. Steve McClaren, slightly different.

'I think he, certainly during the second half of his reign, wasn't happy with a lot of the coverage and I think that he recognised quite early on that the problem at Newcastle United is that nobody speaks and it's left down to the manager and he's left trying to answer questions that he can't really give the answer to and so everything he says then gets picked out and he gets portrayed as Mike Ashley's man.

'In terms of players, some of them are a lot easier to speak to than others. *"A lot of them,"* I think, *"don't even read the coverage so aren't really bothered by it but there are some who claim to not read it, but take a bit of an issue."* I think some of the players do feel that sometimes some of their qualities and talents aren't portrayed as much as they feel it should be and I can understand that to a degree as well.

'In terms of administrators, I don't think they're ever happy with the coverage and I know for a fact they weren't happy with the coverage during Rafa Benitez's final few months but the point I made to them at the time and the point that I would continue to make is that the problem there is it was very one-sided in terms of the coverage but that's because only one side would speak.

'This is something Newcastle United just don't get, and don't understand, is that if you want your side reflected then you have to be more open than they are and nobody would speak on or off the record the last summer before Rafa Benitez left.

'The only story we were getting was from the Benitez side and Newcastle kept on saying it wasn't balanced at all but we asked Newcastle United about these things countless times and they wouldn't say anything. That's their problem. They feel things had been portrayed far too negatively.

'They didn't think there was enough made of the success of getting them out of the Championship which I think is unfair on the coverage. I think the coverage was praiseworthy and yes, maybe it did focus more on Rafa Benitez and the players, but the fact was that the Newcastle United administrators were culpable in getting Newcastle United relegated in the first place.

'So, a slap on the back for getting them back to where most people thought they should have been I don't think was necessarily there,' said Waugh.

Later in this book, I shall share the story with you of how I was approached by a veteran journalist who called my line of questioning "disgusting" after I called out the Golden Lions rugby coach after he claimed his men would give the British and Irish Lions a "hiding".

Salguero accepted that controversial clashes were part and parcel of the competitive sports reporting scene, 'I've never had them tell me a question I've asked is disgusting or rude or anything of that nature. I've seen what I thought were inappropriate questions but you know what, we live in America and people have the right to say what they want to say, and ask what they want to ask and we have freedom of the press here and so therefore, it is what it is.

'You grin and bear it and you accept the good and the bad. However, have I had people who I've asked questions to who have been upset with the line of questioning? Of course, because you have to understand, a lot of the times, this is their livelihood.

'We're covering games and those games represent work, a life, a way to feed a family, so therefore, they take it very seriously. I take it very seriously too because this is how I feed my family. There was one in 2018 where the Dolphins had a quarterback named Ryan Tannehill and he was in his seventh year with the team and the fan base was still waiting for him to become great or to become what they call a franchise quarterback.

'Someone you can count on to compete at a level consistent enough and good enough that you can compete for a championship. Tannehill, frankly, had never done that. In 2016, he was injured. He injured his knee at the end of the season. In 2017, he re-injured the same knee and was out the entire season.

'In 2018, he started out pretty good. The team started out 3-0 and then he got hurt. He hurt his shoulder and he was out for a while. Someone at some point asked Adam Gase, who was the head coach at the time, "So it's Year Seven, your quarterback has never really been all that and now he's hurt a lot. What's the ceiling on him?"

'And Gase said something like if you look at the first three games this year, you have to say that the ceiling is very high and he was playing pretty great and you know, you have to stay with him. And the facts didn't back that up because I had the stats and I had seen the games, I have eyes, and I told him that's not right.

'He was doing okay, and the team won, but the passes he was throwing were unremarkable. He threw three touchdown passes in what they call shovel passes, or flip passes, where the quarterback catches the football and throws it up in the air and a guy that's running diagonally across catches it out of the air.

'It's typically a seven or eight-yard gain. The Dolphins players had turned it into 60 and 50-yard touchdowns and Tannehill gets credited for throwing a 60-yard touchdown on something that you and I could have caught thrown up in the air and the guy catches it as he's whizzing by.

'So, I said to him, his stats are the same as they've always been. In fact, some of them are lower and I outlined 'em to him during a press conference and he got upset. He got angry because his agenda is to lift up his player and make his player feel good about himself so that next week when he plays, he has a certain confidence about him and perhaps with that extra confidence he'll play better.

'My agenda is to tell you what happened and the truth. I'm not there to babysit a player's confidence. I'm not there to hold him up and say it's really, really good when it's really, really average so we have competing agendas and his is psychological and in-house and mine is outside and the truth.

'We went back and forth. It was uncomfortable. He yelled at me. Whatever. That's fine but you know what, Adam Gase is my favourite coach that I've covered during my years at the Dolphins outside of maybe Don Shula, so it was fine. We talked about it later down the road. It was fine afterward but look, it's never gonna be that we're all on the same side.

'I'm on the side of "what happened". If you're awesome, I'm gonna be sounding like a cheerleader and if you're terrible I'm gonna be your worst nightmare because I'm gonna explain to people why you're terrible and lay out, paint the picture of "You're terrible". It's as simple as that and that sometimes grates on people.'

Waugh was not called out, but he had some friction with Steve McClaren when Newcastle were struggling in and around the relegation zone of the Premier League. He recalled, 'I always got along okay with Steve McClaren but there came a point where I felt that some of the questioning probably wasn't strong enough particularly at away games.

'Away matches are slightly different because although there may be another local reporter there, a lot of the journalists are covering from a national point of view and haven't dealt with McClaren so they may just ask the same questions that have been asked the previous weeks and don't necessarily push him and there had been almost the same answer week after week.

'There was a period around Christmas through to January where Newcastle were playing reasonably well and McClaren kept making that point but they weren't picking up any points and they were losing games. I remember it was Watford away for Newcastle twice in two weeks.

'They lost in the FA Cup and they lost in the league and after the league defeat, McClaren started saying the same answer in response to how they played and I just said, "Steve, I'm sorry but you can't give the same answer again. The fans deserve to hear far more than that and maybe you can't give them it, but it's reached a point whereby it is just the same soundbite every week and it's meaningless. Your team can be playing well but they're in the bottom three and it's actually more worrying they're playing well and not picking up points".

'McClaren actually ruffled his hair and said, "I know Chris, but I don't know what else I can say at this stage". Over the course of the next few weeks, I was just a lot more blunt with the questions and eventually it didn't go particularly well and it blew up in a press conference which wasn't my doing, let me just add.

'So there's been a few instances like that where you just feel that some of the questioning on occasions can be a little bit cosy from a local point of view and to be honest when Rafa Benitez was in charge I probably didn't pose as many questions as maybe I should have done.

'Benitez wielded quite a lot of power and had that sort of respect and maybe I didn't push him when there were certain things I really wasn't comfortable with. Certainly, FA Cup selection I think Benitez got away with one to a certain degree.

'I did ask him but I don't think I probably pushed him as hard as I should have done and there were circumstances and reasons behind why his FA Cup selection were as they were but if it had been any other Newcastle United manager that would have put out some of the teams that he did, over the course of the last decade then they would have been heavily criticised, and he probably wasn't heavily criticised as much as he should have been.

'I do think there is also a balancing with Bruce this season (2019/20). I think sometimes questions have needed to be asked but also sometimes it's reached a point where there is too much negativity and that's partly reflected because supporters aren't happy but context needs to be given in these situations.

'Bruce inherited a difficult situation. It wasn't his own doing and he hasn't helped himself with a lot of the things he's said. At the same time, there's this idea that Newcastle should be higher than 13th, well that's their average position under Mike Ashley so they've just had another average season.

'That's not where any Newcastle United fan wants them to be but that doesn't mean the reality of the situation is different. I think for a local reporter it can be difficult sometimes to strike that balance. I, myself, have been guilty of going too far one way or the other on occasion but now I'm more conscious of that, I reflect on that, and try and learn from those situations.'

When I worked at eNCA as a sports reporter, I had a few heated exchanges with South Africa's the then-national football team coach Pitso Mosimane. It started when he accused me of misquoting him in a television report. I still have no idea how someone can be misquoted in an audio-visual soundbite but nevertheless, he believed I had an agenda against him and so he became very confrontational at press conferences.

That was until he failed to qualify for the Africa Cup of Nations, after misunderstanding the rules. Mosimane thought a draw in the final qualifying game against Sierra Leone would be enough to secure qualification but they actually needed to win. He was not immediately fired but suddenly the under-pressure coach's attitude towards me became considerably friendlier.

A few months later at a press conference, before the formalities began, he greeted me with a big smile and an enthusiastic, 'I saw you on the TV the other night.' I smiled, greeted him back, and joked about thinking it was only my mother who watched. Shortly thereafter, Mosimane was axed by the South African Football Association.

I had enjoyed excellent relationships with other players, coaches and administrators. For every Mosimane or Hans Coetzee (more on the Lions rugby coach later, I promise), you will deal with several great people.

Hopefully, you have a clearer idea now of what it can be like covering your hometown team. The key is to step away from being a fan. Take off your supporter cap and be the objective, no-nonsense sports reporter your audience deserve. The fans are ultimately the ones you are representing.

If the coach does not like you, so what? Chances are high that one year down the line, the coach would have been sacked and could even be working elsewhere but you would still be there.

Chapter Four
What Type of Journalist Are You Going to Be?

What type of journalist do you want to be? No, I am not asking if you want to be a sports reporter or a business correspondent, I am talking about your own personal style. A good idea is to attempt to emulate a respected figure in the industry while you hone your own skills and craft your personal style.

It will likely take years, possibly decades, before you are the finished article, but it would only take months, weeks in some instances, for you to craft your style. If for example, you intended to be a hard-hitting questioner, then it would not take you a decade to develop that trait.

It is something that will become part of your repertoire early on. The mastering of that skill is what will take longer. While this chapter has reporters in mind specifically, please do not be discouraged from reading this part of the book if you intend to become a director, producer or graphic artist for example.

Chances are quite high that at some stage in your career, you might be required to conduct an interview and there are tips in this chapter that may assist you further down the line. For example, there are television news channels that will sometimes only send a cameraman to a story.

The theory is that the pictures trump any interviews, but it has been known to happen that an important figure relevant to the story could be present and the cameraman was then asked to conduct an interview. Imagine being sent to shoot the latest construction pictures of Real Madrid's new training ground and Carlo Ancelotti pitches up.

Believe me when I tell you, the bosses back at the office will not care that you were not a reporter, they will only care if you interviewed him or not. Since you will be expected to do this, why not do it well? Be excellent.

In other cases, because resources are often scarce, a cameraman may be sent to shoot an interview with a pre-selected list of questions from a producer or an editor. Alternatively, you might be a junior producer who aspires to one day become a reporter.

Maybe you have decided that you would look into improving your interviewing skills at a later stage but then suddenly one of the reporters calls in sick and you are thrust into the position of interviewing an important player, coach or administrator. Best you be prepared.

The worst kind of reporter is the fan with a laptop. In the old days, they were referred to as fans with typewriters. Possibly in years to come, they may be called fans with iPads, fans with smart phones, or fans with headsets! Who knows for sure, but I am sure you get the point.

A reporter friend of mine at SABC, Velile Mnyandu, once told me that we were all fans ultimately. We grew up watching and loving sport. Of course, we are fans. In fact, it is because we are fans that we became sports journalists in the first place. Velile is quite right.

The important thing to remember is that when the day comes that you interview your favourite player or cover your favourite team, it is crucial that you take off your supporter's hat and don your professional cap. You can celebrate or lament the result afterwards in the privacy of your own home. Objectivity is crucial.

Think of it like this: You are representing the fans. If your favourite football team has just lost 5-0, the supporters are angry. They want to know how this could have happened to their team. They want to know where it all went wrong. They want to know how the coach intends on fixing things ahead of the next match. They might even want to know if the chairman has run out of patience and whether the coach's position has become untenable.

You as the journalist covering the team are obligated to ask those questions and acquire that information on behalf of the fans.

Thankfully, I found it reasonably easy in my first job as a sports reporter proper. I was still in Cape Town covering the teams I loved and supported as a boy. Western Province, the Stormers, the Cape Cobras and Ajax Cape Town (now Cape Town Spurs) were still my beloved teams, but I made a point of leaving my personal feelings aside when interviewing the players, coaches and administrators.

I was easily able to be objective but then it became even easier as I moved to Johannesburg where I covered rugby teams the Lions and Bulls, cricket teams the Lions and Titans, and many of the country's most popular football teams like Kaizer Chiefs, Orlando Pirates and Mamelodi Sundowns, for example.

The advantage I had as a Capetonian, and supporter of Cape teams, was that I genuinely did not care if any of the Johannesburg, or Pretoria, teams won or lost. It was the easiest thing in the world to be neutral. Another advantage I had over my peers was that because I was so emotionally detached, I would ask questions some would not dare ask, whether out of fear of upsetting their favourite teams and players, or a general lack of courage, or who knows what other reason.

In the previous chapter, I briefly touched on an incident between myself and a coach that occurred in 2009 when the British and Irish Lions rugby team were touring South Africa. Well, here it is. A Lions rugby tour takes place every four years but they rotate between Australia, New Zealand and South Africa, so they visit each country only once every 12 years.

In rugby, it is a pretty big deal and a very special tour. Before playing three Test matches against the national team, the Springboks, the Lions played several warm-up matches against the local teams. Johannesburg's rugby team, the Golden Lions, were to be the next opponent for the tourists on a Wednesday night.

The Monday morning prior to the match, the local Lions announced a change in coach. Eugene Eloff had been replaced by Hans Coetzee after a poor showing in the southern hemisphere's transnational franchise competition, the Super 14. Coetzee was in his early 60s at the time and had no previous top-level coaching experience. He had only ever coached high school and age-group level rugby.

I interviewed Coetzee on the morning of his unveiling. The interview was conducted in a respectful manner. I had no reason to be hostile towards him and asked him what he hoped he and his players could achieve against the touring Lions, given that they had just had a poor Super 14 and he would have so little time to work with his new players.

Coetzee confidently told me that his Golden Lions would give the British and Irish Lions a hiding. It was a great soundbite for the evening news and that was exactly what we ended up airing that Monday evening.

Fast forward to the Wednesday night and the overseas Lions annihilated the local pack 74-10. Even if you do not understand rugby's scoring system, you can deduct that that was hardly a flattering score line. At the post-match press conference, I reminded him of his words on the Monday morning and asked him what his thoughts were now.

My follow-up question was about how this level of rugby compared to schoolboy rugby and how much better the British and Irish Lions were compared to the high school teams he had previously encountered. He answered grumpily but what happened after the press conference was truly astonishing.

A veteran newspaper reporter came up to me and asked me what I thought I was doing. He asked me what else I expected the coach to say in that interview on Monday morning and he told me he thought my line of questioning was disgusting.

It genuinely rattled me. Here I was, a mid-20s junior reporter (even though bizarrely, my title was senior sports reporter) doing what I thought a journalist was supposed to do; asking the tough questions and holding people accountable, and I had been hounded out by someone vastly more experienced than myself.

Did I do the wrong thing? Was I out of line? Upon leaving the stadium, I asked my cameraman colleague what his thoughts were about what had happened. He backed me and quoted our channel's slogan at the time, 'No fear, no favour.'

However, that was not enough to put me at ease. That evening, I slept uneasily. While tossing and turning in bed, I could not shake what that veteran reporter had said to me and I genuinely doubted myself. The next morning, I brought it up with my sports editor.

Not only did he back me but he commended me for being the only reporter in that press conference brave enough to ask the questions that rightly should have been asked. The next time the Golden Lions had a press conference, my colleague was covering it and Coetzee refused to speak to her because she was "from eTV and that's where that rude boy is from". She managed to win him over with some sweet talk thankfully.

It first dawned on me in the aftermath of that incident that my true role was to represent the fans. If I was a Lions supporter and my team had just been thrashed 74-10, I would be angry. I would want to know who this clown coach was. I would want to know why he said we were going to give our more illustrious opponents a hiding, but instead the tables were turned in the harshest of manners.

When you are out there in the field as a reporter, remember you are representing the fans. You are in a position to ask the questions that are on their minds. It is a privileged position.

About 18 months later, I had another run-in with a high-profile coach. After the 2010 FIFA World Cup in South Africa, the host nation's assistant coach Pitso Mosimane was promoted to the top job. His first match was a friendly against Ghana and I was covering his press conferences in the days leading up to the match.

As he was new and very few people knew what his tactical approach was going to be, I decided to ask him about his strategy for the fixture. I specifically asked him if he had decided on what formation he would use in this match. He answered that he had not yet determined what system he would employ but he was satisfied that he had sufficient versatility within the squad that would give him several options.

That seemed like a very sensible answer to me, even an impressive position of envy for most coaches, and I eventually used it in my package for that night's news broadcast.

The following morning, I received a phone call from the team's media manager who informed me that the coach was very angry with my report and felt that I had misquoted him to make him look as if he did not know what he was doing. That incident was in 2010 and more than a decade later, I am still at a loss to explain how anyone can be misquoted in a television interview.

Unfortunately, Mosimane and I then had a few unfortunate duels at press conferences where he accused me of "curveball questions" and coming to press conferences with an agenda. He could not have been more wrong. Although I was doing my best to be objective and leave my personal feelings aside, privately I was hoping that Mosimane would do well because if he did well that meant that South Africa's national team would be doing well too.

As it turned out, Mosimane failed in his first assignment to qualify for the 2012 Africa Cup of Nations and was sacked after less than two years in the job. He has since redeemed himself as a club coach in South Africa where he has won the Premiership, several domestic cup titles and the African Champions League with Mamelodi Sundowns. Mosimane had also tasted similar success with Egyptian super club Al Ahly in the ensuing years.

If there was one thing my exchanges with Coetzee and Mosimane taught me, it is that I am personally uncomfortable with hostile interviews. Yes, I was clearly capable of handling them, but it was not something that comes naturally to me.

Later in this book when we discuss dealing with difficult editors and managers, I shall expand on the four core personality types as per the *Flag Page*. For now, I can tell you that the theory argues that there are four personality types and we all have one of these as our primary personality with another featuring strongly as a secondary personality.

They are categorised as nationalities: Control Country, Fun Country, Peace Country and Perfect Country. Put another way, we are talking about control freaks, class clowns, peacekeepers and perfectionists. I, myself hail from Peace Country with a second citizenship from Fun Country, but more on that in Chapter Ten.

By now, I hope you have decided that you will not be a fan with a laptop, but what kind of a journalist are you going to be? It is imperative that you are someone who takes care in gathering information and keeping confidentiality with your sources. These are things that will be taught to you at university or college (hopefully).

The art of conducting an interview is a skill that is not easily taught in my opinion. It takes a lot of work and practice crafting your skills. As a teenager, I wrote for my high school's newspaper and conducted my first interview in that environment but interviewing the school's top academic achiever or a teacher is not the same as interviewing a corrupt sporting administrator.

Nevertheless, any experience in interviewing will stand you in good stead. There are generally two types of interviews: Calm and hostile. In the case of the former, this would be when you interview a player who has just achieved something of significance, like Cristiano Ronaldo scoring his 100th goal for Portugal or perhaps he is back in training after coming back from a long-term injury.

As you can see, there is no reason for this kind of interview to be of a hostile nature. There is nothing controversial to discuss in most cases in these types of interviews.

However, if you are interviewing an administrator who had been accused of money laundering or bribery, then you had best fasten your seatbelt. It is doubly important to have your facts in order ahead of one of these interviews. Politicians, which as we have previously established is what administrators are, are skilled at deflecting attention and for giving elaborate answers to questions without actually answering what you asked them.

There is absolutely nothing wrong with you interrupting them mid-sentence to point out that they are not actually answering the question that you have asked them. Yes, sometimes they may want to give you some background information that will ultimately qualify their answer, and there is nothing wrong with that, but do not let them get away without actually answering your question.

Things can become quite heated in a hostile interview and chances are the controversial figure you are interviewing has previous experience in a hostile interview environment. Make sure that you are excellently prepared and depending on your personality and your comfort, feel free to engage, or disengage, in the hostilities.

Some journalists love sparring with their interviewees. I want to discuss three journalists now who are skilled at mixing things up: Debora Patta, Tim Sebastian and Mehdi Hasan.

Debora Patta was the head of news when I first joined e News Channel in September 2008. She had established a reputation as a hard-hitting journalist who took no prisoners in her interviews, to the point where some may have believed her to intimidate her interviewees.

Patta was certainly not afraid to be confrontational if she deemed it necessary. She hosted a popular investigative journalism programme on e's terrestrial channel, eTV, called 3rd Degree where any guest knew they could expect to be asked the hard questions.

Patta's work had gained her sufficient fame to the point where she had her own Wikipedia page. As we have briefly touched on, Wikipedia is never to be regarded as a source but instead is acceptable for guideline purposes. I perused Patta's Wikipedia page and can say I certainly agreed with the description of her as "direct, to the point and unafraid".

To back that up, consider these two quotes:

"South Africans know her best as the hard-core investigative reporter who ruthlessly rips into everyone from crooked cabinet ministers to medical doctors on the take." Louise Liebenberg, *The Herald*.

"Patta has been called names and is often described as aggressive, but it doesn't seem to bother her much." Bongiwe Khumalo, *Times Live*.

Patta herself has said of criticism of her reporting, 'That means I am doing my job well' and 'we are doing this because we have a true democracy.'[53]

If you would like to get a closer look at Debora Patta's interviewing style, you can search for her on YouTube. There are plenty of uploads. I would suggest you look for a clip where she is physically in studio conducting an interview to get the best idea of how she goes about her craft. You might want to emulate her approach as an interviewer.

Tim Sebastian first came to my attention as the host of the BBC programme *HARD talk,* where he came across as a no-nonsense interviewer who was out to uncover the truth and would not let any slippery politician off the hook. Sebastian is held in high regard in journalism circles and has interviewed U.S. presidents Jimmy Carter, Bill Clinton and Donald Trump.

Although Trump was still many years away from the oval office, as well as South Africa's Nobel peace prize winner, the late Archbishop Desmond Tutu, and the last leader of the Union of Soviet Socialist Republics (USSR), the late Mikhail Gorbachëv.

Sebastian has had several memorable exchanges with corrupt politicians. The wife of former Serbian president Slobadan Milosevic, Mirjana, accused him of being like a policeman and unchivalrous while refusing to answer a question she did not like. This is the kind of hostile reception you can expect in a tough interview environment.

Remember that even though you are unlikely to interview presidents or prime ministers, sportsmen and women, coaches and, especially, administrators are not above the law and as we established in Chapter Two, are among the slipperiest of characters who take advantage of a lack of political savvy or medical, legal and/or scientific knowledge on the part of reporters in the sporting fraternity.

Even though you are a sports journalist, you need to adopt the same approach as your peers in current affairs would. Journalism is journalism whether it is politics, law, business, medical, science and technology, weather or sport.

Hasan, the youngest of the trio I am discussing here, is equally formidable as an interviewer. He was briefly mentioned in the previous chapter and I would recommend you watch his *Head To Head* and *Up Front* programmes on Al Jazeera if you can.

---

[53] Wikipedia. (2022). Debora Patta. [online] Available at: https://en.wikipedia.org/wiki/Debora_Patta [Accessed 28 May 2020].

Hasan always had his facts in order and was able to counter false claims and ask great follow-up questions because he had done his homework properly. No one could ever accuse Mehdi Hasan of not being fully prepared. For this reason, if I was a media consultant to a corrupt politician, I would highly recommend avoiding an interview with him wherever possible.

A former South African deputy president, Baleka Mbete, had rings run around her in an interview with Hasan. It is true that perhaps at times the interview came across as framed in a particular way to portray Mbete as someone who was not doing enough but despite the opportunity to defend herself, she was unable to come away from the interview with her reputation any richer.

For Mbete, the Hasan interview was a public relations disaster. Was Hasan deliberate? Was Hasan wrong? Did he step over the line? Some might feel that was the case, but the reality is that he did not ask her anything, or bring up anything, that was not legitimate.

The public deserved to know, and Hasan made sure they knew while offering Mbete the opportunity to respond. Hasan's style might not be suited to everybody; you can watch some of his exchanges on YouTube, but it is a style that works for him and has proven effective.

There may be a cultural disconnect in terms of approaches between the United States and United Kingdom. He said, 'Most people ask the question and move on whether they get an answer or not. I don't.'[54] Regardless of whether you want to be a hard-hitting, ruthless, griller of an interviewer or whether you prefer a softer approach, the Hasan philosophy of not moving on when the subject dodges your question is a sound policy you should adopt.

An excellent example of the meticulous preparation Hasan does paying off in an interview situation is in his *Upfront* interview with Dr Shashi Tharoor, the former Indian foreign minister. Each time Tharoor attempted to deflect or present facts not relevant to the question, Hasan corrected him, brought him back to the original question and held him accountable.

Tharoor eventually accused Hasan of framing the interview as per a certain agenda that made it impossible for him to give a fair account. In terms of criticism, it is important for you to remember that no matter how determined you

----

[54] The Guardian. (2020). Mehdi Hasan: 'Most people ask the question and move on. I don't.' [online] Available at: https://www.theguardian.com/tv-and-radio/2020/mar/27/mehdi-hasan-interview.

are to prevent your subject from avoiding answering your questions, it is important to give them a fair opportunity to present their side of the argument.

Put another way, if they are guilty, allow them to dig a hole for themselves and then allow them to dig ever deeper while you continue to go about searching for the truth. You will get there eventually, I promise. To get a brief idea of how Hasan goes about his business, and some of the hostile pushbacks he gets from his interviewees, there is a nice highlights reel on YouTube that you can go watch.

The URL is: https://www.youtube.com/watch?v=meUJ2is7gp0

Hasan has had his critics though and just to prove the power and impartiality of the media, I am lifting a criticism of him, from an article on AlJazeera.com. Why not, hey? In a 2019 web article critiquing Hasan's interview with U.S. businessman, ex-navy SEAL and former CEO and chairman of military company Blackwater, Erik Prince, Deborah Avant wrote, 'Hasan's style of questioning was so focused on that "got you" moment, though, that he left important questions about other issues unasked.'[55]

Your main take away from that is that no matter what you do, regardless of your style, you will never please everyone. Decide on what your style is going to be, craft it, hone your skills, tweak it wherever necessary and then confidently back yourself and be true to yourself. Further to that, you will want to be flexible enough to make changes wherever necessary in order to always be on top of your game.

Another attribute that Patta, Sebastian and Hasan all have in common is that they are multi-skilled. They are not just tough reporters who do not shy away from asking the hard questions. They are also skilled as television producers, have held editorial positions in some cases, and have authored books. In a later chapter, we shall look at the importance of being multi-skilled and how it will stand you in good stead but more on that later.

Apart from university degrees and the ability to speak languages other than their mother tongue, there is something else this trio have in common: Trouble. The truth is that when you establish a reputation as a journalist who will not stop in the quest to discover the truth, you could expect all kinds of nasty things to come your way.

---

[55] Avant, D. (n.d.). On how Mehdi Hasan caught Erik Prince in a lie. [online] www.aljazeera.com. Available at: https://www.aljazeera.com/indepth/opinion/mehdi-hasan-caught-erik-prince-lie-190315125456331.html [Accessed 28 May 2020].

In the case of Patta, she had been accused of racism and even received hate mail. Sebastian was expelled from the old USSR in the early 1980s and Hasan had been accused of homophobia, antisemitism and bigotry. I would go so far as to argue that you are not a real journalist until you have been made to feel uncomfortable by those who do not like what you are reporting.

Think back to me lying in bed unable to sleep, virtually broken out in a cold sweat, the night the Golden Lions lost to the British and Irish Lions, in a panic over whether or not I had done my job correctly.

However, I do not want you to come away from this chapter thinking that unless you experience regular sleepless nights, you are not a real reporter. There are other ways to go about your craft. You do not need to be a hard-hitting Patta, Sebastian or Hasan-type. Even in the case of Sebastian, he was not a brutal hard-hitting questioner all of the time.

I would recommend you watch his 1998 interview with Trump; it is on YouTube. In this interview, he was not aggressive in any way whatsoever but managed to extract information from Trump in an excellent manner. He asked Trump all the questions that one would expect him to ask at that time and this is the key, asked superb follow-up questions.

Follow-up questions are almost always unscripted and are only asked as a consequence of what your subject has said. That makes it so crucial for you to listen attentively to what your interviewee is saying. The late, great Larry King, the blueprint master interviewer in my view, said the key to a great interview was listening to what your subject had to say.

Treat your one-on-one interviews as a conversation, especially if it is live or recorded television or radio. People tuning in are watching or listening to a conversation at the end of the day. Make it a memorable conversation.

Preparing is vital but there is no point going into an interview with 10 pre-determined questions and just asking them from one to 10. You would naturally start with Question One but if your subject says something that does not square with the next question, you need to be flexible enough, and indeed alert, to move to the next question, or ask a different question.

This might be a simple example but in 2016, the famous South African cricketer Mark Boucher, who had retired four years earlier, embarked on a coaching career. Boucher was moving from his home in Cape Town to Pretoria where he would be coaching the Titans.

I interviewed him for my podcast and asked him about the move. He mentioned that his dog had made the move too. Quick as a flash, I asked him for the name and breed of his dog. Boucher told me it was a golden retriever named Vegas. My next question was to ask him about the origin of the dog's name.

He went on to share a delightful anecdote of how his friends had hoped to have his bachelor's party in Las Vegas and by naming the dog Vegas, they hoped to plant a seed in the mind of his fiancée, who Boucher believed was unlikely to approve the bachelor's party in Sin City.

There was nothing hard-hitting about that interview. It was all about a former cricketer turning to coaching and how he hoped things would turn out, but by extracting that little bit of fun information out of him, I was able to give listeners of the podcast some insight into Boucher's personal life and it turned out to be a popular segment of the interview.

As it turns out, fans love finding out more about their favourite players' personal lives. If you can find out what car they drive, which neighbourhood they live in, their girlfriend or wife's name, dog's name and so on, go ahead and find a way to build it into your story. Even though it is ancillary information, it is the kind of thing that adds colour to your story and can help breathe life into a potentially boring story about a former player becoming a coach.

Over the years, I have worked on changing my approach from a more confrontational style to one that suits my personality better. Maybe when I was in my 20s, I was more of a firebrand but I have matured since. The point is that I am being true to my own personality. That is what you want to do. Be yourself because no one can be better at being you than you.

Authenticity is everything. Readers, listeners, and especially viewers will pick up on a false façade on your part. Unless being confrontational and brutal like Patta comes naturally to you, it is best to go with a more modest approach. That does not mean letting the villains off the hook. Far from it. Instead, I would advocate for your own customised approach.

As you now know in my early days as a reporter, I was a little more confrontational and succeeded in rubbing up men like Hans Coetzee and Pitso Mosimane the wrong way. Whether or not that was the correct approach is debatable but even now a decade or more later, I am in no doubt that the questions I asked were the correct ones and if the situations were to repeat themselves, I would not hesitate to ask those same questions again.

Remember as a sports reporter, you are there to represent the fans, ask questions on their behalf and report the news to help them better understand the circumstances around their favourite sport, team, players and coaches.

Granted, a press conference is not the same as a one-on-one interview and in the former, you might only have the opportunity to ask one question. In fact, in some cases, a media liaison may only allow you one question or ignore you completely if you have a reputation for asking questions they do not like.

While it is regrettable that your access is cut off to a degree in that instance, do not be disheartened. If a sports team or federation sees you as the kind of journalist, they would prefer not to be asking questions at their press conferences then you should consider that a badge of honour, much like the late Andrew Jennings with the IOC and FIFA.

Remember that in a few years' time, the coach will change, the CEO will change, the chairman will change and/or the sponsors will change but you will still be there. Do not be discouraged. Keep fighting that good fight.

Now let us imagine you are interviewing a coach after his team has just experienced a hiding in an important match. The players did not play well. His tactics were clearly wrong for this particular opponent. The fans are angry and now you find yourself in a one-on-one interview scenario.

You can go the Patta or Hasan route, and be brutal, hard-hitting, in-your-face and grill the coach. Never forget that there is a fine line between being tough and being rude. Do not cross that line. You are not a personal enemy of whoever you are interviewing. You are objective.

The fact that the team just lost should not matter to you. Instead, you are there to get answers. There is also the possibility that the coach, or whoever you are interviewing, is very upset after the defeat and is in a bad mood and could potentially take it out on you, regardless of how tough your line of questioning is.

Even the decorated German coach, Jurgen Klopp, famous for his friendly, relaxed and personable style, has had a go at reporters in the past. They may even deliberately try to bait you. Do not fall into the trap. Avoid that territory like the plague. Instead see it as your chance to show your class and keep calm.

The alternative to the Patta or Hasan approach, is the Sebastian technique as seen in his interview with Donald Trump. This can also be thought of as the Larry King style and is the approach that comes most naturally to me. After playing the harsh questioner with Coetzee and Mosimane, I realised that even though the questions were the right ones, my tone and approach were not really in line with my own personality.

I could not continue to go out there daily as a reporter putting on a performance. I am not an actor. The tough guy persona is best left to the Pattas and Hasans of this world. Instead, I crafted a style that was in line with my own personality and suited me best. Let me give you an example.

A few years after the Lions v Lions fiasco, I found myself in a similar situation. Although many of the players from the 2009 episode were no longer there and there had been at least two changes of coach since Coetzee, I was interviewing the Golden Lions captain (not the same person as in 2009) in a live television broadcast.

They had again lost badly and missed out on the opportunity to reach the next round of an important competition, even though much was expected of them. My question to the Lions captain went something like this, 'There's a big Lions fan sitting at home right now. He is angry after what happened in the last match. What would you say to that guy?'

By framing my question like that, I ensured that the captain could take no offence at all to me. After all, I was asking him to respond to a hypothetical supporter. Moreover, the question was in fact no different to, "You were badly beaten in the last game and fell horribly short of expectations. What do you have to say for yourself?"

The only difference was that the former was a more diplomatic way to ask the question and in doing so, I succeeded in not getting the captain's back up against the wall and by keeping him a little more relaxed and calm, he spoke more candidly and opened up more than he might have done otherwise, I believe. In the end, I was able to conduct a high-quality interview with him. Had the interview been more hostile, perhaps he would not have been so forthcoming with honest answers.

This does not mean that I have suddenly gone soft. Certainly not. If a harsher tone is required, then I shall not hesitate to go there. What you do not want to allow is yourself to be pushed around or bullied by your interviewee. At one stage in my career, I was filling in as a prime time news anchor and while interviewing a high-profile politician, I had to interrupt him mid-sentence because he was veering away from the question I asked.

I simply interjected and said, 'Excuse me but that is not actually what I asked you.' I then repeated the original question. It was not necessary to be combative, but it was important that I was firm and that he knew that I was not going to allow him to get away with not answering the question. Remember being tough and firm does not have to be equal to being combative or rude.

Thus, my preferred approach is to keep things civil and diplomatic and I shall only harshen my tone when I deem it necessary. If you are from Peace Country, you can ask the same tough questions and get to the truth just as Debora Patta or Mehdi Hasan do. Your method will just be different and there is nothing wrong with that.

Patta and Hasan are successful because their interviewing style works for them. They are being true to their personalities. Similarly, Tim Sebastian and Larry King have enjoyed great success as interviewers because their approaches work for them. Work out what works for you, make sure it is in tune with your personality, and you will ultimately be successful too.

Chapter Five
The Various Media Platforms

In this chapter, we shall explore the different platforms on which you will be able to practice sports journalism as well as cast our magnifying glass upon the brave new world of digital journalism. Up until about a century ago, newspapers were king and virtually the only place where you could practice your craft as a journalist.

Forerunners of the modern newspaper included the Acta diurna ("daily acts") of ancient Rome, which posted announcements of political and social events. Manuscript newsletters circulated in the late Middle Ages by various international traders and in England, the printed news book or news pamphlet usually related a single topical event such as a battle, disaster, or public celebration.

The earliest known example is an eyewitness account of the English victory over the Scots at the Battle of Flodden (1513). Other forerunners include the town crier and ballads and broadsides.

Early in the 20th century, the number of American papers reached a peak with more than 2,000 dailies and 14,000 weeklies. That number declined thereafter, though total circulation rose and later, a dozen large chains would gain control of more than half of the American dailies. A pattern of consolidation and merger was seen worldwide though, especially in the second half of the 20th century.[56]

Radio would become the next platform for reporters and then a few decades later, television would join the fray. Some might argue that in the era of network news, television is king but that is not necessarily the case. There was even a song by The Buggles called *Video Killed The Radio Star*.

---

[56] newspaper | History & Facts. (2019). In: Encyclopædia Britannica. [online] Available at: https://www.britannica.com/topic/newspaper.

British pop star, Robbie Williams named his 2009 album *Reality Killed The Video Star*, possibly in the hope of being credited as a sort of soothsayer, at best, or, at worst, as the author of a future popular phrase. Some might argue that digital has killed the video star, or several stars for that matter. The argument has merit, but it is not entirely true.

The world is changing at a frantic pace. What may have been an accepted method today, might be completely outdated tomorrow. It is a case of "adapt or die" and this certainly extends to the world of journalism. The arrival of a new medium brings with it deep suspicion and also dismissal in some quarters. As it turned out, those who dismissed the internet were wrong and many have been predicting the death of radio for decades and yet it is still here.

An argument could be made that digital will be next to rule the media landscape, if it is not already at the top. If in doubt, consider the alleged influence Facebook has on U.S. elections. Even so, with the advent of the internet came the opportunity for news houses to expand.

Some simply copy and paste their print stories on to their websites (not necessarily a bad idea) while others put unique content on their websites and some, but not all, charge a small subscription fee to access that unique online content.

The New York Times falls into that latter category for example and it has proven successful for them. They allow you to read five free articles per month before you have to start paying. Furthermore, and almost certainly because of *The New York Times'* success, other newspapers have put up paywalls on their websites.

The Washington Post, *Miami Herald* and *The Daily Telegraph* in the United Kingdom come to mind, while *The Guardian*, highly regarded for its web content, provides free access but at the end of each article, requests a donation. In South Africa, *The Daily Maverick* follows the same model and this has proven successful for them.

The expectation is that donations coupled with advertising revenues as well as the elimination of printing and distribution costs will more than make up for the loss in subscription fees.

There are advantages and disadvantages no matter what you do. For example, a friend of mine enjoys reading sports articles in his native language Afrikaans on *Netwerk24*. In the past, he has sent me links to articles he thinks I might find interesting. However, as I am not a *Netwerk24* subscriber, I am unable to access the content.

My only option is to subscribe, something that I lack an appetite for since similar content is usually available on other online platforms for free in English, my mother tongue. The strategy of allowing users to read a few articles per month for free on their website before asking for a subscription seems fair enough, especially for someone like me who might only check in to *The New York Times'* website a handful of times per month at most.

The New York Times is widely regarded as one of the best newspapers in the world, although that reputation is up for debate and not just because of the contents of tweets sent by a certain former U.S. president. Later in this book, I shall share a resignation letter from that publication that will challenge your thinking on this famous newspaper.

Nevertheless, given their reputation, why would anyone not want to access their world-famous content? There is no easy answer but let us say hypothetically that you are a fan of American football team the Miami Dolphins. Where do you suppose you are more likely to access better Dolphins content: *The New York Times* or *Miami Herald*?

The answer really should be the latter. Different news houses have different specialities. If I was living in New York and wanted Yankees, Mets, Rangers, Islanders, Giants, Jets, Knicks or Brooklyn Nets content, then of course I would prefer *The New York Times*, or *New York Post*. The same would apply if I was a New York native living somewhere else, or even just an out-of-town supporter of one of these teams.

The reality is that each news media house will have to decide for themselves what their preferred business model is going to be when it comes to their websites. When I joined Al Jazeera, I found myself thrust into an environment where I needed a better knowledge of U.S. sports.

Growing up in South Africa, I had been fed a sports diet of football, cricket, rugby, boxing, tennis, and motor sport mostly. From my point of view, American football, basketball, baseball and ice hockey were games played by those in the United States exclusively.

There is a small and loyal following of basketball in South Africa but considering the time difference(games often only tip off at two in the morning South African time), it really does take a diehard loyalist to follow the NBA.

However, an Al Jazeera sports journalist is expected to know about the NBA, NFL, MLB and NHL. Let me share my strategy with you. I decided that it would be more fun if I had some skin in the game. I had two options. Firstly, I could become more involved in sports betting or secondly, I could pick a team to support and closely follow their fortunes.

Option One was a non-starter for me. Years ago, I was a keen gambler but learnt my lesson when I lost more than ZAR4000 on a Super 14 rugby match. The Sharks, who were top of the standings after seven wins in their opening eight games, were playing the Cheetahs, who were bottom of the table and without a win. I thought it was a sure thing.

Imagine my deteriorating mental condition as the Cheetahs took the lead and then built on their advantage as the match clock ticked on. As their lead gradually increased, so too did my anguish. In the end, it was not even close as the Cheetahs eased to a convincing 31-6 victory.

That was the end of the Sharks as they lost three of their last four games to slip out of play-off contention. It was also the end of my gambling career. In those days, I was agnostic and have since become a Christian, so my conscience prevents me from indulging in gambling now anyway. Given the Sharks-Cheetahs experience, I would say that is a good thing, for sure.

With that option for "skin in the game" eliminated, I picked the alternative, choosing teams to support. It may interest you to know that I picked the Dolphins as my American football team and the Houston Rockets as my basketball team. As I write this, I have not yet visited Miami or Houston and the only reason behind choosing these teams was an affinity for their names.

Dolphins happen to be my favourite marine animal while I think "Rockets" is the perfect name for a team coming out of Houston, the home of NASA. For the record, I thought the Diamondbacks were an excellent name choice for a team playing out of Arizona.

I was also influenced after reading Jerry Colangelo's book *How You Play The Game*, a read I highly recommend to anyone interested in the business around sport. I was close to picking the D-backs, but since I have a phobia for snakes, I picked the Los Angeles Dodgers as my baseball team.

The next step was to select outlets where I would get regular Dolphins, Rockets and Dodgers news. I selected the *Miami Herald, Houston Chronicle* and *Los Angeles Times* websites. I made a point of popping in on a daily basis and this was how I began to learn more about the teams, players, coaches, general managers, owners as well as the leagues, divisions, conferences and history.

Imagine my horror one January morning when I clicked on my bookmarked *Miami Herald* icon to find that the site had suddenly put up a paywall. I am not against any media house trying to make some money. It is crucial in most instances. The problem I had with this was that firstly it had been freely accessible for many years and secondly, I was just a casual fan trying to get some Dolphins information.

I was not interested in reading daily about Miamian politics, business, law, entertainment and arts. Instead of paying, I found myself an alternative website: *Bleacher Report*, a place where the important news surrounding a team or topic is gathered in one place for you to access. I now go to *Bleacher Report* for my U.S. sports news and information in addition to *ESPN*'s website.

You may feel differently and be of the opinion that it is essential for you to subscribe to one of these websites with a paywall in order to access the news that you need. I think if I was a Miamian, Houstonian or Angelino, I would feel very differently and instead be a keen subscriber. Everyone has to make the decision that lines up best with their needs.

In terms of websites that require a subscription to gain access to their content, I would highly recommend *The Athletic*, especially if you are following North American sports. *The Athletic* consists mostly of in-depth, insightful long form content as well as podcasts.

They promise to provide "in-depth sports stories you won't find anywhere else"[57]. At the time of writing, a monthly subscription cost $9.99 per month or an even better $4.99 per month if you commit to a year's subscription. If you are slightly unsure, you can also sign up a free one-week subscription.

Before I move on, I have to share another strategy with you on how you can educate yourself on a sport or team that you are unfamiliar with. A former colleague of mine, Lenn Moleko, had landed himself a job in radio as a sports reporter. The sports editor handed him a golf assignment one day.

Somewhat embarrassed, Lenn approached the editor and explained that he did not know much about golf and asked if he could be assigned a different story. The sports editor, to his credit, relieved Lenn of the golf assignment but made it very clear that he had best brush up on his golf knowledge as soon as possible because his excuse would not be acceptable next time.

---

[57] The Athletic. (2019). The Athletic. [online] Available at: https://theathletic.com/.

This happened to be on a Friday and after work, Lenn made his way to a games store and bought himself the *Tiger Woods PGA Tour* PlayStation game. Lenn spent the entire weekend at home playing *Tiger Woods PGA Tour* and as a result, became familiar with the sport. Maybe Lenn's approach is one that might work for you as well.

One of the advantages of newspapers, radio and television is that they can all have a digital platform too, whereas a blog, vlog, podcast or YouTube show is already a digital platform. It is not however uncommon for a popular blogger, vlogger, podcast or YouTube host to be invited to anchor a news programme on radio or television, or to write a column in a newspaper or magazine.

In many markets, newspapers enjoy a legacy advantage over their rivals from other platforms. Just like a British athlete is more likely to grant an interview to the BBC ahead of NDTV (New Delhi TV), so too in some cases, a player or coach may be more likely to grant an interview to *The New York Times* ahead of a Kansas City local radio station, even if the latter has more listeners than the newspaper has readers.

It is all about perspective in those cases. In many South African markets, coaches hold smaller local newspapers in higher regard than national television or radio stations. It is not always like that, but I would like you to be mindful of this.

One of the disadvantages newspapers have is that they are printed periodically. Some publish two editions per day, others one a day, and others maybe once a week. Sunday-only edition newspapers have traditionally been a big deal.

I remember as a boy my father would return from the shop on a Sunday morning with two of the big weekly newspapers: the *Sunday Argus* and *Rapport*. The latter is an Afrikaans Sunday newspaper and reading it greatly helped me improve my Afrikaans vocabulary and reading skills, although not sufficiently enough to want to pay to read *Netwerk24* articles.

The *Sunday Argus* was an extension of the weekly *Cape Argus* newspaper; one of Cape Town's biggest publications.

Another major disadvantage of a newspaper is that in the modern context when news breaks, it is only possible for a newspaper to bring that story to you whenever their next edition is published. That could be later in the day, tomorrow morning, Sunday or next week. The exception to this is when newspapers are breaking the news themselves.

One attempt to negate this disadvantage is to publish a breaking story on their website, or push the story on social media, usually via Twitter, and promise more details in their next edition. Newspapers will generally excel when it comes to anticipating news. Often, a newspaper article might run with a report that says the coach or the club president is going to resign, or be fired, or a club is planning to make a bid for a player.

However, if an important player suffers a bad injury during training, a radio station can broadcast it immediately. Television can follow a similar strategy to that of radio but the newspaper might only be able to cover that story on their back page (or front page depending on how important sport is viewed by the editor) at a later stage.

Unfortunately, as a rule, newspaper sales numbers have been dwindling for many years. As a result, there is volatility in terms of job security. If you are a junior reporter at a newspaper and there is economic pressure and a decision is taken to cut jobs, you might well find yourself in the firing line. It could be a case of "last in, first out".

The flip side of that is that sometimes management will decide to cut costs by aiming for the top. That makes experienced reporters, who are usually on much higher salaries compared to their junior counterparts, especially vulnerable. The culling of older, experienced journalists has been referred to as the "juniorisation of the newsroom".

In my opinion, it is a mistake because there is much value to be gained from having more experienced staff around. A price cannot be put on the mentoring role they can play but that is not the way management, more concerned with balancing budgets, see things.

We have already discussed the advantage of radio in terms of its immediacy. If a story can be confirmed, radio has the ability to broadcast it immediately. This dynamism makes radio a powerful platform. I have heard over the last decade how radio is a dying medium. The argument is that digital products like iTunes, Spotify, podcasts and online radio will replace traditional radio.

I strongly disagree. Radio has withstood the onslaught, real or imagined, from television and podcasts. It could be the case that radio's market share shrinks, much like newspapers, but like their printing counterparts, I believe radio will still be with us for a long time to come. There is more than enough space in the market for radio and podcasts.

A century ago, listeners had to endure AM (amplitude modulation) broadcasting before a breakthrough of note was made by the introduction of FM (frequency modulation) broadcasting. When FM came along in the 1930s, that should have been the death knell of AM.

Digital audio broadcasting (DAB) was introduced in 1998 and that should have ended FM. Digital signals provide much higher quality and while digital radio mondiale (DRM) offers a higher spectral efficiency replacement for legacy AM and FM broadcasting, the fact of the matter is that AM and FM are still with us.

While that may be surprising, the reality is that CDs and DVDs are also still around despite superior technology being available. Once upon a time, my DVD collection was a personal source of pride. I hopped on board the bandwagon in the early 2010s and gradually began replacing my DVDs with Blu-Rays but then when 4K was introduced, I just drew a line in the sand.

Thankfully for someone like me, there are now vast digital libraries available on video-on-demand (VOD) platforms. Video killed the radio star, they said (or sang!), but the radio star is still with us, so he is not truly dead, is he?

As a journalist, a career in radio offers several options. You can work as a reporter, news reader (or anchor), producer or newsgatherer. This is not limited to news and information radio stations. Most music radio stations also have a news department, although it tends to be considerably smaller than a dedicated news radio station.

In my home country South Africa, there are four different kinds of radio stations. These are community, commercial, public broadcast services and retail. It would be a good idea for you to familiarise yourself with the different kinds of radio stations in your country, if you are considering a career in radio.

Similarly, this list generally applies to newspapers and television too. Newspapers in South Africa fall into the community or commercial categories while television stations can be community, commercial or public broadcast services. I have written articles for community and commercial newspapers.

Commercial newspapers, like all other commercial media, exist to make a profit and those who find employment there can expect to receive a salary. However, this is not the case in community media. I wrote regular rugby, cricket and football world cup articles for the *Worcester Standard*; a community newspaper in the town of Worcester about 100 kilometres north of Cape Town between 2007 and 2010.

I received compensation for these pieces until they changed news editors and the new person in charge was not interested in receiving any written work from me. During that period, I had also moved from Cape Town to Johannesburg and approached one of the local community newspapers, the *Randburg Sun*, with a view to writing for them.

They were happy to publish my writing, but they did not pay their writers. At that stage of my career, I felt I no longer needed exposure and experience. I needed money, so I politely declined.

Radio has the same dynamic in terms of community and commercial radio. When I was at Radio KC, I did so as a volunteer, although they did eventually pay me "petrol money" because I was working too many hours a week at the station to be legally considered a volunteer.

When I moved to P4 (Heart 104.9), I had joined the ranks of commercial radio. It should not come as a surprise to you that it is a significant shift in terms of quality, efficiency and professionalism. Community radio is generally a place for passionate and ambitious amateurs while commercial radio is a place for professionals.

That said, an amateur should not be confused for a novice. Rugby fans will do well to remember that Gareth Edwards, Willie John McBride, Frik Du Preez and Grant Fox were all amateurs. While many people in community media are starting out and learning their way, there are a lot of people present with valuable experience and life skills. Do not underestimate the learning possibilities at a community media house.

A public broadcast service is a grey area in the South African context. Officially public broadcast services are radio stations owned by the national broadcaster, South African Broadcast Corporation (SABC) but the radio stations that fall under the SABC's umbrella are extremely varied. South Africa has 11 official languages and each language has its own dedicated radio station.

For example, Ukhozi FM is the Zulu language radio station and Umhlobo Wenene FM caters to speakers of the Xhosa language. These language radio stations tend to broadcast nationwide. As per the Independent Communications Authority of South Africa (ICASA), a community radio station is a non-profit organisation that broadcasts content that binds a community together.

The criteria that defines a community in this case ranges from language and religion to geography for example. Thus, Ukhozi and Umhlobo Wenene would qualify as community radio stations yet they are public broadcast services. Radio

KC, where I worked in Paarl, is a geographical community radio station offering content that is of interest to the people of Paarl and surrounding towns but not a public broadcast service.

SABC also has SAFM in its stable. SAFM is a talk radio station that to the ear sounds suspiciously similar to commercial talk radio stations like 702, Cape Talk and Power FM. Can you see why I said there was some grey area when it comes to defining a public broadcast service in South Africa?

Other SABC radio stations include 5FM and Good Hope FM. These two are contemporary music radio stations targeting mostly high school, college and university students. To the ear, they sound exactly like any other commercial music radio station in the country. The country's other well-known youth radio station, YFM, is a commercial radio station.

In my opinion, it is farcical to justify 5FM and Good Hope FM as public broadcast services when there is no notable difference when compared to private commercial broadcasters. They are public broadcast services in name only. YFM has to sell advertising to survive whereas 5FM and Good Hope FM enjoy the security of the SABC umbrella.

Retail radio is a little trickier if you are an aspiring journalist. It is specifically designed to improve the in-store shopper experience and bring special offers and discounts to the attention of customers. As you can tell, it is hardly the ideal space for a journalist to operate in but there are opportunities that can present themselves from time to time.

For example, I had maintained a great relationship with the retail radio station where I once worked as a music and entertainment presenter and as a result, they called on me every time there was a major sports event to provide reports and analysis.

These days, radio can also be found on digital platforms and this has opened the market greatly. It also means though that you or your radio station could easily be lost in the crowd. That is the disadvantage and the same is true of podcasts.

There are millions of podcasts now available on iTunes and other platforms. Finding one that you enjoy listening to is surely an exercise in trial and error but at the same time, it might not actually be humanly possible to listen to all of them, even in your preferred category.

It is therefore critical to stand out if you are thinking of starting your own podcast. One tactic that works for some podcasters is to tie it in with a media house that is already well established. If your podcast is linked to *The Guardian* newspaper for example, then you can benefit from having it promoted via their platform which is likely bigger than yours, especially if you are just starting out.

I would recommend the book *Contagious* by Jonah Berger. Your idea or product must contain six core principles, according to Berger. The first is social currency in the sense that people like to appear smart when they talk about it or share it. Secondly, it needs to trigger. Think of the idea behind "top of mind leads to tip of tongue".

The third principle is emotion. You want to kindle an emotional fire, be it positive or negative. A world cup victory is as effective as Sepp Blatter being done for bribery and corruption. There is a human tendency to imitate popular habits. If it is easy to imitate, it is more likely to become popular.

Think of a silly little dance video that has gone viral. This is the fourth principle. Next is practical value. You want content that is useful to people. Finally, people do not just want to share information, they like to tell stories. Make sure your content is able to travel under the guise of idle chatter.[58]

It might not always be possible to incorporate all six of these principles in your content but strive to get as close as you possibly can to boost your chances.

In terms of emotions, positive arousals include awe, excitement and amusement or humour. Negative arousals include anger and anxiety.[59] Those are the emotions you are aiming for to help make your content go viral. Contentment or sadness does not create the same kind of internal stir.

The goal is to aim for high arousal emotions. People are more likely to share content that they care about, makes them look good, and is currently relevant and unique.

These are some of the things to consider if you are hoping to become a broadcast journalist and hoping to expand into the world of podcasts or media entrepreneurship, which is something that we shall cover later in this book.

Television in South Africa is also regulated by ICASA. Much like newspapers and radio, community television stations exist to focus on local matters. For example, there is Cape TV, Bay TV, 1KZN, Soweto TV and GauTV

---

[58] Berger, J. (2014). Contagious: how to build word of mouth in the digital age. London: Simon & Schuster. pp. 22-25

[59] Berger, J. (2014). Contagious: how to build word of mouth in the digital age. London: Simon & Schuster. p. 109

which covers Cape Town, Gqeberha (formerly Port Elizabeth), KwaZulu-Natal, Soweto and Gauteng respectively.

Thanks to frequency overflows, it is possible to watch Soweto TV even if you are outside of the famous Johannesburg township. I used to live in Randburg, roughly 25 kilometres north of Soweto and it was possible to watch Soweto TV on my television in my living room.

That said many of the community television stations in South Africa have joined the country's top satellite television platform, DSTV, so you could be in Cape Town and watch Soweto TV now. By being on the DSTV platform, the community television channels are guaranteed a fixed income from the satellite company Multi Choice.

This income is often what is needed just to stay afloat. What saddens me is the content on many of these community channels. In theory, they should be focused on local programming and news. For example, if a new set of traffic lights has been erected on a busy road, or there was a robbery of a community tuck shop, then it needs to be broadcast on these platforms.

These channels generally lack the resources to put together such content anyway and have resorted to programming featuring American pastors. It provides them with much needed income, make no mistake, but it defeats the object of a community television station in my opinion.

Televangelists make for great Sunday content but when they dominate the airwaves from Monday to Friday, can you really call yourself Soweto TV, Cape TV or Bay TV?

That said the last time I had the opportunity to tune in, Bay TV and 1KZN particularly impressed me with their evening news offerings. It was very clear that an effort was made in bringing their viewers high quality local news. Well done to the decision makers at those channels.

If you are an aspiring sports reporter or anchor, these community television channels are exactly the kinds of places where you can gain invaluable experience and screen time that might be unavailable to you at a bigger network. You do not want to stay in community television for too many years though.

Often, the positions are voluntary without compensation, but if you are unable to afford university fees to acquire a journalism degree, then I think community media is an excellent alternative choice. Often, you will learn practical skills that are not being taught at tertiary institutions.

I would advise you to check your country's local broadcast regulator to find out what different broadcasting categories there are where you live. In the United States, they have the Federal Communications Commission (FCC). The FCC regulates interstate and international communications by radio, television, wire, satellite, and cable in all 50 states.[60]

Do some research and find out who your ICASA or FCC is. It may be that you have a regulator that plays the same role or maybe where you live, the communications authority has a very different model.

Let us now look at digital journalism platforms. There are so many these days, but the main ones would be websites, blogs, podcasts and vlogs. It is ever-evolving and for that reason, I am not going to even attempt to define it outside of it being journalism in any form that is web-based.

The reality is that by the time you read this, there may well be something new on the scene. Embrace it regardless of your personal feelings. That will give you longevity.

Moreover, I am not going to teach you how to produce a podcast or YouTube video. This is something that you should learn at university and besides, the point of this book is to equip you with the information you did not receive in tertiary education. Besides, if you did not receive these teachings as part of your education, there are several free resources available, aptly on YouTube itself.

Generally, journalists who go the digital route are doing so as freelancers or entrepreneurs and while I have dedicated chapters in this book to freelancers and entrepreneurship, I would like to discuss these elements briefly here.

A journalist can have their own website where they promote their past work. Most reporters and presenters do this. Believe it or not, many companies are opposed to their journalists doing this but the great irony is that often before hiring a presenter, and often reporters, producers and video editors too, they would ask their candidates to provide them with a show reel or demo of their previous work.

I wonder from where they think these candidates acquire the content for their show reels and demos. You can also use a social media website like LinkedIn to promote yourself. Further to that, links to your previous work can also be especially helpful when other media houses are looking for an expert opinion.

---

[60] Federal Communications Commission. (2017). What We Do. [online] Available at: https://www.fcc.gov/about-fcc/what-we-do.

101

Your website can aid you in being found. These days, Twitter would play a similar role.

In February 2013, South Africa was rocked by the news that one of its darling athletes, the amputee sprinter Oscar Pistorius, had been accused of murdering his girlfriend. During the Pistorius murder trial in South Africa, my colleague Michael Appel impressed so much with his reporting that he received a telephone call from Sky News asking him to do an interview with them on the trial.

Michael was able to grow his profile this way and he was also contacted by other international broadcasters during the court case. Radio reporter for 702's *Eye Witness News* Barry Bateman became a Twitter superstar in an instant when *Match Of The Day* host Gary Linekar sent a tweet identifying Barry as the authority on all things Oscar Pistorius.

Linekar enjoys great prominence in the United Kingdom, not only as a former prolific striker for England but also now as a television personality where he is currently the highest paid on-air personality at the BBC.[61] So much so that one tweet by him promoting your work, can launch you into significant prominence. Maybe I should add a chapter to this book, *How To Get Gary Linekar To Tweet About You.*

If your reporting is noticed, it can elevate you to a position where other news outlets are keen to have you on their channels as a guest. Now in the case of Michael Appel, his then employer would have had no problem with him appearing on Sky News, provided Sky introduced him as a reporter from that particular media house, but they would not have felt as obliging had it been a local rival like eNCA for example.

Similarly, if they did have the audacity to ask Michael to appear on their channel, it would have been foolish of him to agree. It is worth noting that Michael has since worked at eNCA before moving into the digital space and then taking a job at Al Jazeera himself. While the additional exposure is great, be mindful of where your bread is buttered.

If you are working at a local television news channel in the Republic of Ireland and CNN calls to invite you to be a guest on their channel, there is nothing wrong with asking them to introduce you as a reporter from the channel where you currently work.

---

[61] The Independent. (2019). Gary Lineker volunteers to cut down £1.75m BBC salary. [online] Available at: https://www.independent.co.uk/arts-entertainment/tv/news/gary-lineker-bbc-salary-match-of-the-day-a9108286.html [Accessed 29 May 2020].

Digital journalists have the advantage of not being tied down in that way. If you are able to gain a reputation as an authority on a particular subject, there would be no reason why you could not appear on Sky News, BBC, CNN and Al Jazeera all on the same day.

Further to that, imagine the exposure you would get not only for yourself but also your business. You could be introduced as "John Beresford from The John Beresford Show". That would be a double whammy in your favour.

There is another type of digital journalism which Yusuf Omar describes as "wearable journalism". Omar is the co-founder of *Seen* (previously *Hashtag Our Stories),* a video publisher that has trained more than 3,000 people in over 104 countries to tell their stories with their phones.

'We felt traditional media was out of touch with real people and real stories. They didn't think Donald Trump was going to win the elections. They didn't think Brexit was going to happen in the UK. We felt that was because we were speaking to politicians and pundits and experts and commentators, and not people on the ground.

'If we could train people to tell their own stories, we'd get access to a new type of video content. We also raised the issue on constructive journalism; there's a problem in society and here's somebody making it better with solutions which of course you see in sport all the time; rags to riches stories. People kind of becoming heroes, or even unsung heroes in terms of the coaches and the trainers and marginalised communities,' he said.

While the world of digital media, particularly the entrepreneurial side of it, comes across as a world of glamour and freedom, there is a warning that you need to be mindful of. Sadly, no matter how good you are at growing an audience on a digital platform, it can oftentimes be hit and miss.

One of the curses (or blessings depending on how you look at it) of being a broadcaster is that when I watch YouTube videos, I do so with my broadcaster's eye. The number of channels and videos I see that have hundreds of thousands, even millions, of views, likes and subscriptions despite breaking basic video rules is staggering.

There are people who have videos with millions of views, and channels with millions of subscribers who would never get their content beyond the video edit suite at a community television channel. It is tragic, but the reality is that in the digital space quality does not always win the day. The internet is a black hole of content. You could produce the most amazing content, but no one will ever hear it, read it or see it.

I have heard it said that Millennials, loosely defined as those born between 1981 and 1996 and currently the most sought after economic and political demographic, favour content that comes across as more real and less scripted. Omar is unsurprised by this phenomenon, 'I think that the audience have never been more forgiving of shaky, hand-held footage. They really just want a good story.

'I think that's where the emphasis lies, on good story telling. Everything else is a benefit. I think that technology is making a lot of those other processes easier. So, you've got apps that will help you automate video editing and you've got apps that will help you shoot better but the hard bit is how do you tell a good story? How do you identify a good story? How do you discover good stories? And I think that hasn't changed no matter what platform you're on.'

That should fill you with encouragement if you lack confidence in your skills as a videographer, video editor, script writing or even as a presenter.

That is great if you are an entrepreneur or a freelancer, but as an employee, one thing you will constantly be reminded of in a commercial newsroom is to be mindful of your audience. Every commercial media entity exists to make a profit. In order to make a profit, they have to sell their product.

That product is being sold to a specific target market and you will be expected to create content that relates to that target market. If your target audience does not care that your videos are littered with jump cuts, then who are you to argue?

Even so, you still want to keep to the highest standards of quality and be mindful of Berger's six principles to help make your content contagious, while being encouraged by Omar's message that the audience has never been as forgiving of imperfection.

I do want to stress though that imperfection is not a licence to fail to strive for excellence.

While there are examples of overnight success, the truth is it seldom happens that way. It requires a lot of hard work, which in turn produces higher than usual growth. After a nasty falling out with ESPN, Dan Simmons launched the sports media company *The Ringer*. It includes a podcast network of more than 30 shows, a sports news website and a film production unit. In March 2020, Simmons sold the company to Spotify for an initial $155 million.[62]

Simmons, as it turned out, became the first podcaster to make the Forbes Celebrity 100 list.[63]

Yes, that kind of money is alluring and what happened to Simmons is an example of what is possible, but you need to understand that it is the exception rather than the rule. Your goal should be to produce excellent blogs, podcasts and videos. The viewers, subscribers and sponsors will follow.

Your goal should be to make sure that your podcast is available on all the various platforms like iTunes, Google Podcasts and Sound Cloud. Some of them offer free hosting, while others have pricing plans depending on the size of your clip. You can promote your blog, podcast or YouTube channel using other social media platforms and this is generally the way it is done.

In 2019, it was estimated Spotify spent between $400 million and $500 million acquiring other podcast assets. Spotify CEO Daniel Ek said, 'The trend that we are investing in here is that radio is moving online. We bought the next ESPN.'[64]

Sport is a big deal in the digital journalism space. Identical twins, Cory and Coby Cotton teamed up with friends, Cody Jones, Tyler Toney and Garrett Hilbert to start the *Dude Perfect* YouTube channel.[65] It was not necessarily journalistic in nature but combined sport, entertainment and humour. At the time of writing, the *Dude Perfect* channel had 59.2 million subscribers on YouTube.[66]

[62] Forbes. (n.d.). Bill Simmons. [online] Available at:
https://www.forbes.com/profile/bill-simmons/#1ada4e7648ce [Accessed 29 May 2020].

[63] Shapiro, A. (n.d.). Spotify Sale Mints The Ringer's Bill Simmons As Podcasting's First Big-Money Superstar. [online] Forbes. Available at:
https://www.forbes.com/sites/arielshapiro/2020/06/04/spotify-sale-mints-the-ringers-bill-simmons-as-podcastings-first-big-money-superstar/#23fa7e837e52 [Accessed 29 May 2020]

[64] TechCrunch. (n.d.). Spotify is buying The Ringer to boost its sports podcast content. [online] Available at: https://techcrunch.com/2020/02/05/spotify-is-buying-the-ringer-to-boost-its-sports-podcast-content/ [Accessed 29 May 2020].

[65] Dude Perfect Wiki. (n.d.). Cory. [online] Available at:
https://dudeperfect.fandom.com/wiki/Cory_Cotton [Accessed 5 May 2022].

[66] Dude Perfect. (2019). YouTube. Available at:
https://www.youtube.com/user/corycotton.

While the above-mentioned examples are of digital-only media houses, traditional media outlets have also branched out. We have already discussed newspapers offering their content online, for free or otherwise. Similarly, radio and television news stations have websites with blog posts, podcasts and video content.

Often on YouTube, a television channel will have its own channel where it posts selected clips from their live broadcasts. This will usually be in the form of an exclusive interview, feature, or something that was particularly entertaining or interest.

It is almost needless to say, but they all have social media accounts that they use to further promote upcoming content or they might use it as a means to direct traffic to their websites, YouTube channels, podcast platforms or original platform.

ESPN Cricinfo is a website that has seen it all. Launched in 1993, it was intended as an internet hub to unite cricket fans all over the world. All those years ago, Cricinfo was the disrupter but over the decades, the website has had to adapt with the ever-changing landscape in order to remain relevant.

Sambit Bal is the editor-in-chief of ESPN Cricinfo. He says that while the website enjoys a legacy that most sites can only dream of, there can never be any room for complacency, 'Cricinfo invented journalism on the web. That's a big statement to make but in 1993, there wasn't the web as we know it today, so Cricinfo was the first sports content website in the world.

'That's a huge legacy to build on. Cricinfo was born out of passion. It was born out of a need and a desire to connect cricket fans around the world with the game. That's the legacy that we take. That's the founding principle that we carry in our hearts. Digital journalism and digital content is constantly evolving so you have to keep pace with everything that's happening.

'The way content is created, the way it is packaged and the way it is delivered. All those things have changed and all those things change almost every year and today, we not only deliver content on Cricinfo but we deliver the same content on multiple platforms like YouTube, Instagram, Facebook, Twitter, TikTok, or whatever.

'We're constantly innovating. You can say also that Cricinfo was the first website to video stream a cricket match, which was in 1998 but video wasn't an integral part of Cricinfo's package until the early 2000s. Now, we are able to deliver a website that features video, audio, graphics, data, all that put together, and sometimes, it's like running a newspaper, a TV channel, a news station and a data analytics operation at the same time.

'That's the beauty of digital journalism. You can bring all these things together. We carry four different elements. We are constantly evolving but also constantly learning new things. I'm an old print journalist who printed magazines before I came to Cricinfo and you take all those activities that you learnt in journalism.

'I'm glad that I was a journalist when there was only print. All those disciplines in print journalism and the rigours of print journalism, and all the values of print journalism that you bring to a digital platform, you don't sacrifice those elements, but you change the way you write or create content.'

Bal mentioned social media platforms like Facebook, Twitter, Instagram and TikTok. It is true that some journalists have managed to carve a niche for themselves using these platforms too. It is possible to be a "Twitter reporter" but generally the social networks act as supplementary mediums.

In the digital space, you are likely to write a blog post and then promote it via the social media platforms. Sometimes, there can be cross-promotion so you could use Twitter to promote your YouTube video for example. Be flexible, be versatile and constantly be open to innovation, no matter the urge to resist.

It is very important in the modern age to include all the elements, according to Bal. He argues it has to be strategic and appropriate, 'We don't see video as an add-on. You just have to decide which story works best which way. So obviously a match report, or ball-by-ball commentary, or a lengthy piece or feature, will be text but something like an explainer we do on video.

'We don't just do video or audio for the sake of it. Whenever there's a piece of content that comes on our plate, we decide which element of it should go to which medium and then you try to deliver that piece of content in that way. A 3,000-word piece can never be done on video.

'If you write, a think piece takes you an hour or sometimes longer, but if you want to do a quick analysis on something, it is much better done on video because you can just record it and it's done quite quickly. Obviously, you still need the knowledge, but that kind of instant analysis is really good for video.

'Unlike a lot of other people, I don't think text is history or that it has no use. I think every medium is just a way to deliver it, so you need to choose the right message for the right medium.'

The digital sphere has made it possible for anyone to have a platform. That is a good and a bad thing. You might struggle to find work as a journalist but with the help of blogs, podcasts and videos, you can promote yourself to such an extent that it builds a CV or demo tape, which you can use to land a big job.

You might find that your own initiative grows into your own media business. You will read more about that in our chapter on starting your own media business. But what if it is your ambition to work at a place like ESPN Cricinfo and you have heeded the advice to start a podcast or YouTube channel covering cricket.

Does someone like Bal view you as competition? If your quality is not up to scratch, will Spotify ever make you a $155 million offer to buy your fledgling business, as they did in the case of Simmons?

Bal says, 'What modern publishing allows is a lot of content and it's very creative today, compared to a few years ago. With the democratisation of platforms, it has also brought a bit of anarchy. There is a lot of great content on YouTube but there's also a lot of junk. Everybody can be competition, but the challenge is how do you know what is relevant.

'That's the main thing. YouTube is there for entertainment but is YouTube a medium for delivering news and delivering credible analysis or credible voices? That's the challenge. Apart from these voices there's a whole bunch of noise. Anybody with a platform, like someone who is independent and producing content by themselves, struggles for credibility.

'Credibility is built over years and years and years. Who are they accountable to? A media organisation is accountable to its consumers, its readers and there's a reputation to uphold. That's the danger of a lot of people publishing without moderation. Everything that goes up on our site is fact-checked.

'There is a team that is working behind the scenes to make sure that information is credible. That is the way of a media professional. The basic principle of why we became journalists is to serve news and information in a certain way so there are checks and balances.'

Credibility is everything in journalism. People spend years, even decades, establishing a solid reputation but credibility is something that starts with you and therefore, you can build a foundation as soon as you begin. If you are starting a podcast or a YouTube channel, make sure that you hold yourself accountable and uphold a certain universally accepted standard of quality.

People might dismiss you at first and question your credibility but make sure that if they do investigate your affairs, you achieve a clean audit. Over time, it will become noticeable to others. Be patient, work hard and do not compromise but do not be afraid of making mistakes along the way. Remember what Omar said: audiences have never been more forgiving.

A simple Google search will reveal the top sports podcasts and YouTube channels. Do yourself a favour and consume this content. You do not have to subscribe or listen every week but by consuming it, you can get a good sense of how others are going about their business. You can emulate the best bits.

Similarly, look at blog posts. Once upon a time, blog posts were just newspaper articles or opinion pieces on a website. Now, blog posts include pictures, audio and video clips. Digital journalism changes all the time. Stay up to date, embrace it and whatever you do, do it with the highest standards of journalistic integrity.

Chapter Six
What an Aspiring Sports Journalist Should Study

There is a common misperception that you have to have a degree from a top university in order to make it in life. I am going to show you in this chapter that it is about you, the individual, rather than the university, even though there are some exceptions, but that is entirely out of your control.

Consistently ranked as one of the world's richest men, Bill Gates (you may have heard of him) dropped out of Harvard University in his second year. Gates is not the only high-profile former university drop out. Facebook founder, Mark Zuckerberg also left Harvard in his second year, while the man behind Apple, the late Steve Jobs also never completed his university education. Gates and Zuckerberg have since returned to Harvard to receive honorary degrees.

You might read that and think, "Well, if it was good enough for Bill Gates and Mark Zuckerberg, then it is good enough for me. After all, university is rather expensive". Perhaps you may have a point but unless you have a grand plan to start the next super tech company and are supremely confident of becoming a billionaire by the age of 25, then it is best you avoid their example.

I would recommend a university or college degree to any aspiring professional. In years gone by, it was something that commanded respect. These days just about anyone in the office will have one, sometimes two or three, and human resources (HR) and recruitment staff tend to look out for it before selecting potential candidates for a job interview.

You could miss out on a job interview simply because you do not have a tertiary qualification. It is important that you understand that many people in HR and recruitment do not understand the day-to-day activities of the jobs that people at their company are employed to do.

For example, I worked at a channel where the HR staff were more interested in meticulously counting the hours staff were physically present at the office than actual job performance. They were not interested in whether you were performing well in your job, they wanted to know whether or not you arrived on time and did not leave early.

Further to that, they also took great interest in whether or not you took your obligatory lunch hour. Once I asked, hypothetically, what would happen if you were unable to take your lunch hour because it was a busy day filled with breaking news? I was told I had to take my lunch hour.

Seemingly, it was of more importance to spend an hour in the company canteen eating than covering a sports corruption scandal. I wondered if the channel's head of news and CEO would have agreed with that assessment. When you enter the job market, be prepared to encounter HR and recruitment team members who are not familiar with the ins and outs of your job. If you get yourself in that mental headspace now, you can save yourself several headaches down the line.

My own story has a little bit in common with Gates, Jobs and Zuckerberg. No, I am not a tech billionaire, but I did not finish university at the first attempt either. When I started my university career, I did not really know what I was doing. As I was finishing high school, all I knew was that I wanted to be a radio presenter.

What do you study for that? I was a keen listener of 5FM (one of South Africa's national music radio stations). I figured that if I emailed Mark Gillman, the breakfast show host, he might not reply since he was probably a very busy person and might be "too important" to reply to some high school kid. Therefore, I opted to email each of the presenters.

I knew that law of averages would count in my favour and I would have assembled a sample of answers from which to work and then I would be in a position to make a decision. Sure enough, not all of them replied but many of them did.

I was grateful and the main takeaways I got from their replies was that most of the presenters had no qualifications and the job was one that relied on talent more than anything else. You either have it or you do not. I have since come to experience that myself in broadcasting.

I firmly believe that as a television or radio presenter, even if it is news, you have to possess a natural talent or otherwise, it is going to be an uphill struggle for you. I would argue it is easier to host a Top 40 countdown show on MTV than to present a news bulletin.

In the former, you just announce the names of the songs, with a few anecdotes about the artists in between which a producer could research for you. In the case of news, you need that natural ability in front of a camera as well as an excellent general knowledge of current affairs.

I am not saying that an aspiring television or radio news presenter should consider a university degree unnecessary since they have been blessed with a talent. Far from it. There is an old saying that goes, "Hard work beats talent unless talent works hard". Remember that.

After receiving the feedback from the 5FM presenters, I had determined, in my infinite teenaged wisdom that a university degree would be a waste of time. Why spend three or four years on campus when I could just start pursuing a radio presenting career straight out of high school? I did not need a degree anyway.

The 5FM presenters confirmed this. Well that was what I was thinking until I saw a television interview with Robert Marawa, a Metro FM radio and SABC television sports presenter. Marawa was just starting to become popular and was discussing his career. He mentioned to the interviewer that he had a university degree because he wanted credibility and authority when he spoke on air.

That sounded like an excellent philosophy to my ears. Marawa had changed my mind. I decided my new strategy would be to complete a university degree and then become a radio presenter. I had been fascinated by sport and politics since the age of eight and had built up a wealth of knowledge over the years, naturally accompanied by opinions, and if I was going to share those opinions on air, a tertiary degree would give me credibility and authority.

However, as I was finishing high school, I was experiencing a lot of doubt. I did not actually know what degree I wanted to study. It seemed to me that joining a university and studying a random degree for the sake of having one was not wise. I considered taking a gap year and packing fish in Alaska.

That became an attractive option. I could go work in Alaska, earn U.S. dollars, come home after a few months and have more money than all my friends, while figuring out what it was that I was going to study. After all, as I completed high school, the U.S. dollar was trading at ZAR13.53:1, so an Alaskan adventure appeared alluring.

My parents were supportive of my idea although they did nothing to actively support my fish-packing plan. The fish-packing plot was ultimately dead in the water. My indecisive mind wandered away from the icy waters of North America and considered something closer to home.

Instead of attending university, I thought perhaps I could become a real estate agent but my mother was firmly against that. She thought a commission-based career was not a wise choice and to be honest, it was only a brief flirtation anyway.

I decided that since I was so unsure, I would sit out the next year while working out exactly what it was that I wanted to do, and maybe still end up spending six months in Alaska. Make up your mind, kid.

That was until one of my close friends phoned me to tell me he was on his way to Stellenbosch University to sign up and I should join. Clearly, my 18-year-old self was easily swayed; good thing he was not offering drugs, and I hopped in the car with him and we made our way to the university's administration building.

To my credit, I did at least sit with a career counsellor and explained my "Robert Marawa Theory". He recommended a BA degree in something that I honestly cannot even remember but by the time the academic year started, I had altered my choices sufficiently for it to become a BA International Studies.

If that sounds vague to you, imagine what it sounded like to me as the weeks went by and the doubts just increased. I was struggling to work out what exactly the point of this degree was. What was I actually studying towards? Never mind that, the real question was more like, what was I doing? I then began researching an alternative option; something that I believed could be helpful.

I settled on a degree related to information technology but it would alter my programme so much that I would have to wait until the start of the next academic year to start. I explained this to my mother who agreed that I could drop out for the remainder of my first year and resume at the start of the following year.

My father was unimpressed. He said I must "find direction" and while he was right; my life was veering out of control, the truth is I had no direction at all and some six weeks before my 19th birthday, and less than four months into my first year of study, I was a first-year university drop out.

Direction would come in the form of my father. After mucking about for nearly a year after dropping out, he told me to come and work for him. He owned a transport business and while I was no truck driver or mechanic, he handed me an office job with a very fluid job description.

Officially, I was to be a bookkeeper of sorts. I would take care of the wages and in addition to that, I was also a runner. He would send me all over Cape Town to fetch or drop off parts and products. It was a lot of fun to be honest. Many days, I simply lazed about the house with nothing to do but watch television.

Recognising the comfort of my position, I never ever gave my dad any grief. He once phoned me on a Saturday afternoon, about an hour before a Springbok rugby match was about to kick off, asking me to go fetch a part for one of his trucks.

As you can imagine, I had no enthusiasm whatsoever for that task, especially since the location was at least a 45-minute drive away which guaranteed by the time I returned home, the first half would probably have ended. Nevertheless, I bit my lip and did the necessary. After all, I had probably done very little in the previous week (or even fortnight) anyway.

My dad was more serious about this than I was and instructed me to take a short course in accounting. I was never going to resist and made my way to the Cape Peninsula University of Technology. I found a pamphlet for a short course in *Basic Accounting* and out of pure curiosity, I eyed over the other course offerings and there it was, *Introduction to Radio Broadcasting*. I picked it up, drove home and convinced my dad (read mother) to pay for both courses.

The accounting classes took place on Mondays and Wednesdays, while my radio classes were on Tuesdays and Thursdays. The short courses ran from August to late November/early December and when I received my final results, much was confirmed.

I failed *Basic Accounting* and passed *Introduction to Radio Broadcasting* with a distinction. I had not failed my father completely since he still allowed me to work for him as a bookkeeper cum runner, but my future path was now rather obvious. Radio is what I wanted to do, and I had just learnthowto go about doing it too.

After recording a demo, I researched the different community radio stations in Cape Town and the Western Cape province. Community radio plays an integral role in local broadcasting in South Africa and from the perspective of a youngster looking to break into the industry, it was the perfect starting point.

After I phoned all the community radio stations on my short list, there were two who had vacancies, or at the very least were having auditions. The first was Radio KC in Paarl, a town north of Cape Town about 35 kilometres from my parents' house where I was still staying.

In a quirky twist of fate, the other was MFM; Stellenbosch University's campus radio station. Perhaps justifiably some two years after I rejected the university, MFM rejected me while Radio KC gave me a chance.

I was going to host a late morning Saturday show from 11:00 to 13:00. My excitement was only matched by my nervousness. I planned my show out as best I could, selected the songs I wanted to play, packed my bag and drove to Paarl for what would be my first ever radio show. What followed was disastrous.

My introduction link was an abysmal nervous-filled shocker. My second link was not much better and despite being in an air-conditioned studio, I found myself sweating from nervousness as I looked up at the clock. We had been on air for 12 minutes and already my third song was about to end.

What was I going to say at the end of this song? I had prepared but clearly inadequately and then to make matters worse, the station's programme manager, Georgette Frolicks, came barging into the studio. She was not impressed by my introduction either but to her eternal credit, she encouraged, rather than lambasted me.

She reminded me of how excellent I sounded on my demo and that that was the sound she wanted to hear from me. I took a deep breath, gathered my thoughts, and reminded myself that this was my dream and that I was actually sitting in the hot seat. This was my chance to make it and I might not get another opportunity.

The song ended, my microphone was made live by the sound engineer and I began my third link. I cannot remember what I said but I basically started the show over and it was chalk and cheese compared to the drivel I had produced just a few minutes earlier. I was up and running as a radio presenter.

I had overcome my fear and nerves. By the end of the show, I had grown in confidence so much that I could not wait to come back the following week for my second show. Thank you, Georgette for giving me my chance and believing in me.

That was on 20 March 2004 and on 17 June 2005, I was no longer working at Radio KC. I had graduated from Saturdays to the weekday afternoon drive show and then joined commercial radio station P4 (later Heart 104.9) as a sports presenter on their afternoon drive show.

There was no interest in me possessing a university degree from P4. All I had to do to secure the job was do an audition. The news editor, Jan Weintrob handed me a script of an earlier sports bulletin and asked me to present it as if it were on air and after doing just that, I was offered the job on the spot.

I also began working at a retail radio station, Feel Good FM as a weekend presenter; Saturdays and Sundays 11:00 to 14:00. Judy Jegels was the station manager at Feel Good FM and she did not ask me for proof of a university degree either.

In September 2008, I left radio to join e News Channel (later eNCA) as a sports reporter. Admittedly, I was helped in getting the job by a former radio colleague, Robin Adams, but the sports editor at e, Dylan Rogers, also never asked me for evidence of a university degree.

The difference between my radio career and television sojourn was that in the latter, I had worked almost exclusively in journalism whereas in radio, it was on the entertainment side of things. You could argue that in entertainment, a university degree is of less significance than in a more professional journalistic environment.

Nevertheless, Dylan was more than willing to give me a chance and perhaps my lack of a university degree was made up for by my broadcasting experience.

After five years at e News, I joined the fledgling news channel, ANN7. I remember in the interview I was asked if I had a degree. I answered honestly but was also happy to point out that I hoped my experience would negate that. Interestingly, when I joined Al Jazeera, I was not asked about a university qualification. Not at first anyway.

My initial contract with Al Jazeera was as a freelancer. My attitude was that I would take the short-term deal, work really hard to impress the bosses and hopefully, land a full-time job. That was exactly how it worked out but in the separate job interview for full-time employment, the issue of a university degree came up.

To my great relief, I was told by the HR staff member that the channel did not view degrees as obligatory for journalists. I was able to become a full-time employee at Al Jazeera without a university degree but it could have been a very different scenario.

There are many countries that will not even look at you without a university degree in your possession. At one point, I was in early talks with CGTN to join them in Beijing. Nothing came of it, but a Chinese company cannot employ a foreigner who does not have a university degree.

If you have ambitions of working outside of your home country, I would strongly advise completing a degree. It will eliminate a lot of stress and also, more importantly, open doors, or perhaps in some cases, prevent doors from being shut before you even land a job interview.

After those talks with CGTN, I decided that even though I had managed to come this far in my career without a tertiary qualification, not having a degree was limiting my options. I am happy to tell you that in 2019, I graduated from Edinburgh Napier University with a MA International Journalism.

That said please do not think that you need a master's degree in order to land your dream sports journalism job. Certainly not. Similarly, I would prefer you not thinking you have to have a degree from Harvard to stand any chance of finding yourself in that dream job.

My recommended path would be for you to acquire a degree but if you are unable to do that, then either take a short course in journalism or look around your local news media houses to see if there are any job shadowing or internship opportunities.

There is no reason why someone straight out of school cannot join a media house as a runner and gradually work their way up. There is power in simply being available sometimes. As my colleague Andy Richardson once put it, "Half of life is about showing up".

There are two aspects you need to consider now. What are you going to study and where are you going to study it? We shall tackle the former first.

The obvious answer is that you want a degree in journalism. This would usually be a Bachelor of Arts degree, usually from a faculty such as Arts and Humanities but sometimes also social sciences, and typically takes three to four years to complete.

While this is a solid starting point, I think it is worth your while thinking about what kind of reporting you would like to specialise in. In my opinion, there are too many reporters, especially in sport, who lack sufficient knowledge of their subjects, despite their best efforts.

For example, the 2020 Covid-19 global pandemic exposed many reporters for their lack of medical knowledge. This should not come as a surprise since these reporters studied journalism, media, communications, film or something similar in most cases.

In my opinion, the early Covid-19 news coverage was especially poor and it may very well have contributed to the social media wild fire that was spread. The reality is that we live in an era where "Karen from Facebook" and "@Doug452" have become "experts" and for that reason, we need to safeguard more than ever before.

I do not blame the reporters in this instance though. In my experience, oftentimes news editors throw these journalists to the wolves and expect results. You cannot for example, at a minute's notice, send a South African reporter to the United Kingdom to cover a court case.

Why not? Well for starters, British law differs from South African law. Remember, students typically take four years to complete a law degree. Many attorneys that move countries are unable to find work in their new country because they lack sufficient local legal knowledge or their qualification in not recognised.

It is not uncommon to hear stories of lawyers from Eastern Europe moving to Western Europe and having to work menial jobs because they are unable to practice law in their new countries. With that in mind, what chance does a news reporter have of familiarising themselves with the law of a different country in a very short space of time?

Something like this nearly befell me in 2012. I was in London to cover the Olympic Games when a news editor in Johannesburg came up with the idea that since I was in London, it would be a good idea to send me to the High Court to cover the Shrien Dewani case.

If you are not familiar with Dewani, he was accused of plotting his own wife's murder while on honeymoon in Cape Town. He was eventually extradited but for a humble sports reporter such as myself, fully immersed in all things Olympic Games, a change of assignment to the courts of London would have proven nothing short of disastrous.

Thankfully, I had a strong sports editor back home who fought on my behalf and I only gained knowledge of this ludicrous idea upon my return to the country a few weeks later.

Nevertheless, had I been a current affairs or general news reporter that assignment would almost certainly have had my name on it and what would I have done then? While this is specifically a legal example, it could have been true of medicine, science, technology, business or environmental affairs too. This is why I recommend excellent supplementary knowledge for journalists, sport or otherwise.

Perhaps you are thinking that it makes sense for a general news reporter to be equipped with this kind of general knowledge, but sports reporters do not really need that. Not true. Earlier in this book, you read of the skulduggery at FIFA and the IOC. Their administrators ran rings around many sports reporters because of their general lack of knowledge of the law.

This is not meant as a criticism of those reporters. It is just the state of affairs but hopefully, this will help you see how important it is to improve on the status quo in the industry. Most sports reporters can name the starting line-up of a team, or even all the teams in a specific league, but can they name the board members at a sports federation?

What about Lance Armstrong and other dopers? A good knowledge of medicine would come in handy there. The average sports reporter is unlikely to be capable of naming even 10 banned substances as per the World Anti-Doping Agency's banned substances list, let alone explain what they are.

Once again, I am not attacking my colleagues, but merely pointing out that we have been let down by the system and the villains have taken advantage of this. For many years studying journalism was enough but perhaps we should think about studying law, business, medicine, science, technology or something else and then specialise in that field within sports journalism.

I think it would make for more powerful journalism. One of the media's problems is that someone with a law degree working as an attorney is almost always going to earn substantially more money than someone with a law degree working as a journalist.

Similarly, someone with a PhD is going to specialise as a surgeon before they become a medical journalist; unless you are going to be the face of a network news channel as is the case with Dr Sanjay Gupta at CNN. Perhaps the solution could be to study journalism, media, communications or something similar but stack up on books or take short courses dealing with your preferred area of specialisation.

I particularly enjoy the writings of Andrew Jennings and his uncovering of the bad guys at FIFA and the IOC. Some of his work is referenced in this book. If it is something that interests you, go out and get those books and build up your knowledge.

Just before I move on to where you might want to study, I want to discuss briefly media and communications degrees. These days, those degrees could be separate or combined, depending on your institution. They are traditionally distinct from journalism since media and/or communications is directed more towards people seeking a career in public relations or the more technical elements of media like video editing, vision mixing, animation and graphic designing for example.

These days, you might find that some of those are covered in a degree in Film and Television or something similar which is a good idea for someone keen to become a producer or a director for example. These degrees are not to be ruled out. You might not want to be out there in the field firing questions at Gianni Infantino or Thomas Bach, but you have an artistic talent that could be of great value as a graphic designer for example.

You can still work in sports journalism creating beautiful bespoke on-screen graphics. Later in this book, I shall discuss careers in sports journalism other than reporting, because not everyone can be, or wants to be, a reporter.

Looking at the most recent World University Rankings[67] by *The Times Higher Education,* the top 10 was made up of the usual suspects. In order, they are:

1. University of Oxford (UK)
2. California Institute of Technology, or Caltech (USA)
3. Harvard University (USA)
4. Stanford University (USA)
5. Massachusetts Institute of Technology, or M.I.T (USA)
6. University of Cambridge (UK)
7. Princeton University (USA)
8. University of California, Berkeley (USA)
9. Yale University (USA)
10. University of Chicago (USA)

The United States dominates the top 10 with a couple of British universities adding a smidgen of diversity. ETH Zurich breaks the duopoly in 15th place while the Peking University, Tsinghua University (joint-16th and both from China) and

[67] Times Higher Education (THE). (2021). World University Rankings. [online] Available at: https://www.timeshighereducation.com/world-university-rankings/2022/world-ranking#.

the University of Toronto (18th) are the only other institutions in the top 20 outside of the UK and USA.

The American and British domination continues as only the National University of Singapore (20th) and University of Hong Kong (30th) break up the cycle from positions 20 to 30. Germany features in 32nd-place with LMU Munich with Australia's University of Melbourne coming in 33rd place.

The University of Tokyo is 35th while the University of British Columbia (Canada), Technical University of Munich, Karolinska Institute (Sweden), École Polytechnique Fédérale de Lausanne (Switzerland) and Paris Sciences et Lettres-PSL Research University Paris feature in positions 37, 38, 39 and joint 40th respectively.

My home country South Africa does not have a university inside the top 100. The University of Cape Town (UCT) is the highest-ranked South African tertiary institution at joint-183rd.

These are just some selected university rankings for you. Did you see your university's name there? If you did that is great but if not, do not be disheartened.

When I was researching a university degree for myself, my starting point was *The Times Higher Education* World University Rankings. I wanted a degree from one of the world's great tertiary institutions. *How wonderful would it have been to boast a degree from Oxford or Princeton,* I thought. Perhaps you might be thinking along those same lines. Slow down.

The Times Higher Education World University Rankings are judged according to certain performance indicators like the university's teaching, research, citations, international outlook and industry income. You would expect the learning environment to be excellent, but research is judged by three factors: volume, income and reputation.

Citations factor in research influence. Excuse my cynicism but when someone from Oxford makes a statement, it automatically carries more weight than someone from the University of Johannesburg (UJ). That is not taking away from Oxford and its magnificent achievements, but the truth is that Oxford has established an authoritative reputation over a few centuries, and deservedly enjoys that privilege.

That does not however mean that something superb is incapable of emerging from UJ, but it does mean an Oxford paper is more likely to be cited than a UJ paper.

International outlook includes the staff, students and research and industry income factors in knowledge transfer. While I have nothing against the rankings; in fact, I personally cite them, I want to point out that they are more about research, prestige and honour.

Edinburgh Napier University, where I completed my master's degree, is ranked between 501st and 600th (the rankings do not specify an exact ranking position that far down on the list). At worst, I graduated from an institution ranked 600th and at best 501st, but despite that I have managed to land myself a job at Al Jazeera; by most accounts, one of the top television news networks in the world, and do not forget that I did not actually have a degree at the time I joined the channel.

You might say that a channel like Al Jazeera that is based in a country where English is not the first language, needs to lower its entry requirements in order to attract people and that media houses in countries where English is the first language would have higher entry levels. Not true.

I personally know people who work at some of the top television channels in the United States and United Kingdom who have graduated from South African universities like the University of the Witwatersrand (251st-300th), University of KwaZulu-Natal (351st-400th), UJ (601st-800th), Tshwane University of Technology (1001st-1200th) and Rhodes University (not ranked).

Interestingly in South Africa, Rhodes enjoys a reputation for being the number one learning institution for journalism. Imagine you considered the university rankings as the gold standard and discovered Rhodes was not even ranked after completing your degree there. Not to worry, I have friends who graduated from there and they are doing just fine, both in South Africa and internationally.

These people I personally know who graduated from South African universities who are now working at top television news channels are doing so ahead of people who earned their degrees from places such as Duke University and Northwestern University; ranked 23rd and 24th respectively.

Moreover, one of the journalists interviewed for this book studied at the unranked Mary Immaculate College in Limerick and went on to be a key member of production teams at places like Sky Sports and BeIn Sports.

Let me make it very clear, I am not saying the university rankings are of no meaning, or belittling places like Oxford and Princeton. What I am saying is that if it is not possible for you to study at these elite universities, you should not think that your career is over before it even started. There are so many news media houses and you will find one that is willing to give you a chance.

From there, the ball is firmly in your court. I can also tell you that once you have built up sufficient experience and earned a reputation as a journalist, hardly anyone will care where you completed your degree. Having a graduation piece of paper from one of those top universities is prestigious but it is not the be-all and end-all.

If any of this makes you feel slightly uneasy, let me dash your hopes of ever studying journalism, media, communications, film and/or television at Caltech right now. They do not offer those specific degrees. Simply put, they are not that kind of institution.

Caltech describes their core curriculum for undergraduates as one that will equip you with "substantive experience in problem solving, collaboration, and communication".

Further to that, Caltech claims its students will be able to, 'manage increasing academic challenges while developing resilience and confidence, develop and satisfy their intellectual curiosity, collaborate effectively and ethically, recognising diverse models of academic collaboration and communicate to a range of audiences through a variety of media.

'Demonstrate understanding of foundational concepts from the sciences, use disciplinary thinking, analytical skills, and a range of methods in the sciences, apply their knowledge and skills to diverse problems within and across disciplines, significant study in the humanities and social sciences, explore and expand upon learning in fields beyond intended areas of specialisation, appreciate and understand the contributions of the humanities, social sciences, and arts to human endeavours, and engage in informed analysis of cultural, political, and economic issues.'[68]

Looking at that, I would argue that if you are planning a career in science and/or technology, then the California Institute of Technology is the perfect place for you. Why, while writing this, I glanced at their home page and the first three items that caught my eye dealt with science, robots and NASA. If your plan is to study journalism, or a related degree, then Caltech is not for you.

---

[68] Dean of Undergraduate Students. (n.d.). Core Curriculum for Undergraduates. [online] Available at: https://www.deans.caltech.edu/core-curriculum-undergraduates [Accessed 30 May 2020]

Contrastingly, my alma mater features several options if you search for journalism programmes on its website.[69] These are, in no particular order:

1. BA (Hons) Journalism.
2. BA (Hons) Television.
3. BA (Hons) Mass Communications.
4. BA (Hons) Social Sciences.
5. BA (Hons) Photography.

In my home country South Africa, UCT offers *Film and Television Studies* as one of its Bachelor of Arts majors, in addition to *Media and Writing*.[70] According to their website, the major in Film and TV Studies offers "a thorough grounding in the history, theory and analysis of film and TV".

It also encourages "creativity through storyboarding and scriptwriting". UCT says, "The skills provided give students access to careers in academic teaching and scholarship, film journalism, film festival management, and film librarianship".

The wide-ranging knowledge of film also effectively complements creative practice in screenwriting, production and direction, they say.

Interestingly, the major in Media and Writing "weaves together theory and analysis of broadcast and print media with extensive creative practice. Students are trained in writing and editing for a wide range of media: they may specialise in news reporting, investigative journalism, freelancing, sports journalism, advertising, documentary, writing for television (soaps and sitcoms), youth culture and the media, writing for magazines, feature journalism and travel writing".

Now we are talking. As ostensibly unfathomable as it may seem at first, as an aspiring journalist, you would be better off studying at UCT than Caltech. However, if your goal is to become one of the world's leading scientists and discover a cure for HIV, then you would pick Caltech over UCT as a more desirable option.

I mentioned earlier that in my opinion, it would be good for journalists to have supplementary knowledge by way of alternative degrees, diplomas, short

---

[69] Napier. (n.d.). Courses. [online] Available at:
https://www.napier.ac.uk/courses?q=journalism [Accessed 30 May 2020]
[70] www.humanities.uct.ac.za. (n.d.). Degrees & programmes | Faculty of Humanities. [online] Available at: http://www.humanities.uct.ac.za/hum/undergraduate/degrees.

courses and/or extensive private reading. Something that caught my eye on the UCT undergraduate prospectus[71] was the section at the end of each major entitled, "What Can I Do?"

In terms of philosophy, UCT says, 'Philosophy graduates have gone on to work in a variety of areas, occupying posts in: Law (corporate, mediation, prosecution, defence); Computing (artificial intelligence, expert systems design); university or college teaching; senior management; legislative policy; mediation; medical ethics; journalism; film and media.'

This was what the UCT document said about its politics major, 'Typically, our students go on to pursue careers in law, journalism, human rights-related organisations, nongovernmental organisations, government, and the public service, business and research.'

Did you take note of journalism, film and media? Do you see why I recommend this kind of supplementary knowledge even for sports journalists? Someone at UCT clearly agrees with me, "Imagine a job as a professional journalist without knowing the fundamentals about the world of politics; or as a young manager in a large company in South Africa without any prior knowledge about how South Africa became a democracy and how our democratic system works".

Your journalism qualification is important, but the supplementary knowledge is king. If my argument has not convinced, you and you remain determined to obtain your journalism degree from a top-ranked university then by all means go for it, as long as your chosen institution will provide you with the skills you will require when you leave the campus and join the working world.

Ideally, the kinds of skills you will want to have upon graduating would include specialist industry knowledge and experience (more on how to gain that experience later in this book), analytical skills (this is crucial), excellent spoken and written communication (you should ideally already possess this as a raw talent before starting your studies), general research skills and how to find sources.[72]

---

[71] Explore your options for 2018. (n.d.). [online] Available at: http://www.humanities.uct.ac.za/sites/default/files/image_tool/images/2/2018%20UGH um %20EXplo%20web.pdf [Accessed 30 May 2020].

[72] Top Universities. (n.d.). Journalism Degrees. [online] Available at: https://www.topuniversities.com/courses/journalism/guide [Accessed 6 May 2022]

These days, there is more of an emphasis on creativity too and while I like creativity, and think it makes for beautiful writing and designs, your primary goal is to make sure that your writing is factually and grammatically correct. If you are someone who is not naturally creative, do not for one second feel that journalism is not for you. There is a place in this group for you too.

Back to the issue of graduating from one of those elite universities. According to CollegeFactual.com,[73] the top 10 universities for bachelor's degrees in journalism in the United States in 2022 are:

1. Northwestern University.
2. Washington and Lee University.
3. University of Southern California.
4. University of Wisconsin-Madison.
5. The University of Texas at Austin.
6. University of Minnesota-Twin Cities.
7. University of Missouri-Columbia.
8. University of Florida.
9. University of Maryland-College Park.
10. George Washington University.

The University of Florida boasts that some of its graduates have gone on to work at places like *The Washington Post* and *ESPN*; the latter being a dream job for many sports journalists.

I would again say that while that is a wonderful achievement, and source of pride for both university and graduate that does not mean someone who graduated at a supposedly lesser institution cannot find employment at places like *The Washington Post* or *ESPN*.

A colleague and friend of mine graduated from the University of Florida. A proud Gator, I hope she is not too mad at me for that comment.

That said, CollegeFactual.com claims a journalism degree from schools on this elite list typically translates into higher than average income after

---

[73] www.collegefactual.com. (n.d.). 2022 Best Journalism Bachelor's Degree Schools. [online Available at: https://www.collegefactual.com/majors/communication-journalism-media/journalism/rankings/top-ranked/bachelors-degrees/ [Accessed 6 May 2022]

graduation.[74] According to them, a graduate from one of the elite schools typically averages about $6,500 more per annum.

While I would not dispute their findings, in my own personal experience, it has made no difference where someone studied and I cannot stress this enough, if you can afford to go to Northwestern University and graduate with a journalism degree then do it, but if you cannot afford, or cannot travel to one of these top institutions, you should not be discouraged or disheartened.

Look at me, my university is ranked between 501st and 600th in the world and I am doing just fine.

There is another exotic option that may be available to you and that is international study. If you are European or North American, you could go spend a few years studying your degree at the University of Hong Kong for example. Depending on how adventurous you are, an overseas option could be a great experience.

It is true that there are employers that might frown upon a qualification from the University of Hong Kong, particularly in the US, but you need to determine the risks such a choice may or may not present to your career aspirations. In my view, the world is changing and given high university fees and student debt, which has become an electoral issue in many countries, the days of alternative degrees or qualifications could be near, if they are not already with us.

Speaking of a changing world, have you considered acquiring your degree online? It is a magnificent innovation in my view although be warned that some countries, like the United Arab Emirates, do not recognise online degrees.

If you are hoping to land yourself a job in Dubai or Abu Dhabi, an online degree would not be a wise move but having said that, the world is changing all the time and by the time you complete your qualification (or reading this book for that matter), chances are good that the UAE may have decided to recognise online degrees. One of the consequential impacts of Covid-19 may very well be an emphasis, or at least an encouragement, in the area of distance and online studies.

Further to that, there are also several online options these days. One of the best known is The Open University, who purport to be the UK's largest academic institution and a world pioneer in distance learning. While they do not offer a

---

[74] 74 The Best Journalism Schools (2013). The Best Journalism Schools. [online] College Factual. Available at: https://www.collegefactual.com/majors/communication-journalism-media/journalism/rankings/top-ranked/.

specific journalism degree, they do have something that could be of interest to you; a BA (Hons) Arts and Humanities (Creative Writing).[75]

This degree focuses on a range of approaches to writing, helping you develop your writing skills in several genres including fiction, poetry, life writing, and scriptwriting for film, radio and stage, while also helping you develop important skills in complex argument and critical commentary.

In terms of short courses, which you might want to consider to help increase your general knowledge, Udemy and Kajabi are among the best-known but there are several out there, like the fledgling KnowBrainer that offer great value. There is a good chance that several short courses could impress a recruitment officer and even if it does not, it is proof of your own personal self-enrichment.

There are no negatives in that. Many job adverts specify that they would prefer the successful candidate to be a self-starter and/or self-efficient. How much more of a self-starter can you be with several short courses under your belt?

In terms of physical classes, you can enrol in a short course such as those I studied at CPUT, by simply contacting your local learning institutions. I actually returned to CPUT four years after my *Introduction to Radio Broadcasting* course (and insipid *Basic Accounting* non-effort) and completed a short course in *Journalism.*

It may not have been a degree, but it at least gave me some grounding and understanding which would stand me in good stead as I became a sports journalist proper less than a year later when I joined e News. Check with your local learning institutions to see if they offer short courses.

In conclusion, what you want to do is identify a tertiary institution that you can afford to attend. Research and carefully select the degree you want to study; journalism is your likely starting point but think about where you might want to specialise, and then go for it.

Upon completing that degree, consider supplementary short courses; there are many that are online these days as well and build up a personal library on your chosen specialised subject matter. I am a little more old-school, so the books on my bookshelf bring me a sense of pride but you may prefer an e-book library saved in a cloud.

---

[75] The Open University. (n.d.). R14 | BA (Hons) Arts and Humanities (Creative Writing). [online] Available at:
http://www.openuniversity.edu/courses/qualifications/r14-cw [Accessed 30 May 2020].

What you want to do is equip yourself with as much knowledge as possible, so that when you are sent to cover a story, your senses are alert to what is taking place beyond your interview or press conference.

Chapter Seven
Sports Law

No matter what platform you are using to practice your journalism, there are certain dos and don'ts. This could differ from country to country and it is best you familiarise yourself with the law. This is something that is usually easier for a current affairs reporter as they tend to deal with court cases and legal matters more often than a sports reporter.

That said you do not want to be caught out. Imagine being overlooked for an assignment to cover a FIFA corruption court case in favour of a current affairs reporter with little sports knowledge. It might sound wrong, but it happens regularly because news editors generally do not trust sports reporters when "sport becomes news".

Consider the 2014 Oscar Pistorius murder trial. How many sports reporters were covering that event compared to current affairs correspondents? You can quite rightly argue that it was a news story that just happened to feature an athlete and there is merit in that argument.

The other side of that debate is that you could establish yourself as the sports reporter that is assigned these stories. By doing so, you could establish a reputation as the go-to sports reporter, analyst or expert on legal matters involving sportsmen and women.

That kind of reputation would be valuable as a media freelancer or entrepreneur but equally powerful as an employed journalist when it comes to contract or salary negotiations, or even your next job interview.

Bear in mind, there are significant challenges to being a legal expert or authority. Law differs from jurisdiction to jurisdiction. Attorneys can sometimes find themselves out of work when they move to a different country, or they are forced to upskill by way of courses, or sometimes studying a fresh degree, which often might be financially impossible.

It is not unheard of for lawyers to move to a new country and work as taxi drivers because their qualifications are not recognised in their new location.

While the following quote from Heenan Blaikie LLP is not specifically targeted at sports journalists, it certainly applies, 'While very few statutes and regulations are specifically targeted toward sports, sports law is a very real legal discipline, both multi-faceted and extremely specialized.

'Whether the focus is on amateur or professional sports, there is an acute need for legal advice and negotiation skills in this important industry. Sports law requires its practitioners to stay abreast of a quickly evolving universe.'[76]

The average sports journalist is unlikely to ever be an expert in the law, and frankly it should not be expected, but by educating yourself and acquiring this additional knowledge, it can only stand you in good stead. Although this chapter is dealing specifically with the legal side of sport, I would point out that if you are not overly enthusiastic about sports law, then pick another niche wherein you can specialise within sports journalism.

This could be bribery, corruption, doping, injuries and recovery, medicine, racketeering, science, sexual abuse or technology among many other areas. As the saying goes "Knowledge is power", so I would encourage you to try and learn a little bit in each of these areas. Even though you are being encouraged here to specialise, most reporters will be expected to be a jack of all trades, so keep that in mind.

Parliamentarians pass new laws all the time and amend old laws just as often, so you need to stay on top of these things. One great way to do this is by subscribing to the relevant media e-mail lists. Governments and sports federations send out regular press releases and sometimes just by reading through them, you will be able to stay in touch with the latest news.

Oftentimes, the information is not overly newsworthy but by staying up to date, it will almost certainly help you in the future.

For this chapter, I assembled an expert panel of three lawyers who specialise in the sports side of the law. They are Exavier B Pope I, Esquire; a sports legal analyst based in Chicago, host of the #SuitUp podcast, owner of 528 Media and a contributor to Forbes.com.

Larry Fenelon; a partner and founder of Leman Solicitors law firm, specialist sports lawyers based in Dublin. Fenelon acts for a lot of sports governing bodies

---

[76] www.bestlawyers.com. (n.d.). Best Sports Lawyers in Canada. [online] Available at: https://www.bestlawyers.com/canada/sports-law [Accessed 31 May 2020]

and athletes and ancillary organisations involved in sport. Thirdly, we have Andrew Nixon, Head of Sport at Sheridans in London.

Pope, Fenelon and Nixon hail from the United States, Republic of Ireland and United Kingdom respectively. This book would never have been completed if I had attempted to interview sports lawyers in every country on Earth. So, if your country is not listed here, you can contact a sports lawyer in your area and request some relevant reading material.

Further to that, you might want to familiarise yourself with your country's constitution and contact your parliament and request documents and other reading material from the sports portfolio committee, or any similar portfolio grouping.

The discussion began with me asking each of the panel members to define sports law. Pope asserted, 'Sports law is essentially the areas of law that cover what happens in and around sports. I think that we are learning in these modern times that the definition of what constitutes sports law is broader than we thought it was.

'Sports law can be anywhere between what happens in a professional sports league as relates to the playing conditions, or owners versus their players, and that's labour law. There's also arbitration law. It can be about financing a stadium. There's tax and public finance law and how it relates to the individuals that vote in the districts where those stadiums are.

'Now you're looking at politics and legislation and how people vote. You see athletes sticking up for what's happening in communities, so now you're talking about criminal justice reform. So what sports law is, is much bigger than what we see on the field.'

Fenelon added there were many who questioned whether there was even such a thing as sports law. He believes there is. 'It is a mélange of different laws including contracts, constitutional law, practices and procedure, disciplinary systems, sponsorship, commercial and intellectual property.

'Sports law is probably all of that and more. So, yes, there are books and modules at university but basically they're not as binary or singular as contract law or criminal law for example,' he claimed.

Nixon argued that sports law is most definitely a category of its own, 'The first school of thought which I think is the one I subscribe to, is that there is such a thing as sports law on the basis that first of all, there's a genuine and bona fide body of sports law arising from tribunals such as the Court of Arbitration for Sport.

'So, sports law has its own pack of jurisprudence if you like. Secondly, sport is also privately regulated and privately governed. Yes, those private regulations are in essence governed by general law, governed by employment law, governed by the laws of contract and governed by company law in whatever jurisdiction but those private regulations are nevertheless the framework for sports law and the application of those rules and regulations are really the crux of what sports law is about.

'Because of that uniqueness and those nuances, I subscribe to the view that there is such a thing as sports law. That said there are many others who simply take the view that they are general lawyers but working within the sports industry.'

You might come away from reading those definitions thinking that perhaps there is the law, and that sport simply finds its own little space within that. That argument, while having merit, would then also have to render, for example, labour law as a subcategory within the greater legal landscape.

Most people have no problem referring to labour law as a standalone category. It is therefore worthwhile to ask if there is any specific legislation that applies just to sport.

That is not the case in the Republic of Ireland, but Fenelon pointed out, 'There might be sports bodies that were established with statutory footings such as Sport Ireland, which is effectively the purse strings of government to regulate and pay capital and current grants to sports governing bodies but nothing beyond that.

'There's certainly gaming and betting laws but they would not be specific to any particular sport. So, you wouldn't have Irish rugby legislation, you wouldn't have Irish soccer legislation or Irish Gaelic games legislation.'

This was a matter that would differ from country to country as Nixon reflected, 'In France, sport is effectively regulated by the government. It's regulated by the laws of the land. They have something called the Code d'Sport, the code of sport, a civil code which sets out how legislation works and is applied to the sports industry.

'Whereas say in the United Kingdom, sport is entirely private so there's no public interference. There's no governmental interference in the sports industry, or the sports sector. But obviously at the same time, sport still operates through its own set of private rules and regulations whether that be governed by, or regulated by the Football Association, or the Rugby Football Union, or the England and Wales Cricket Board.

'They all have their own private regulatory framework which is obviously capable of being forced and challenged under normal general law but they are still the private laws of that particular sport. Obviously on a broader level, there is 35 years of case law coming out of the Court of Arbitration for Sport and that itself gives the sports industry its own body of law, or its own jurisprudence if you like.

'So, it depends on the jurisdiction, but that kind of case body of law is almost of central importance right across the board.'

Pope offered a more simplified view on laws unique to sport, 'You have plenty of rules, regulations and laws that relate to sport. Think about rules governing safety in a stadium. Think about playing conditions having to be at a certain level of safety to comply with certain laws.

'Think about any park district or the rules and regulations in your town. Sports law can apply to your local park. It can also be fishing and gaming and how that's regulated. Consider how sports law applies to what's happening in gambling; how sports betting is regulated.'

Further to asking the trio of experts about laws specific to sport, I also asked them about sports laws that may be unique to their country. Nixon said every sport had its own peculiar set of rules and regulations, 'I suppose one which is of interest and which I think is unique to the UK is basically the sports industry at an elite level, and at a grassroots level, is largely funded by NGVs who obviously exploit commercial rights and then filter that money down but also a big part of that is public money through bodies called Sport England and UK Sport.

'One of the most interesting things about their role is they fund and invest in sport in the UK but because they hold the purse strings to public funds, they also set certain criteria, which you must meet in order to access the public funds and a lot of that criteria is around good governance, good regulation, having good integrity provision in place, having diverse boards, dealing with safeguarding issues in the right way and they always use that role in holding the purse strings to public funds to make sure sports bodies in particular are well run and fit for purpose so they play a really important role in that respect.

'There's the Institute of Sport in Australia, which obviously played a similar role about 20 years ago but I'm not aware of too many countries around the world akin to Sport England and UK Sport and obviously, bodies that play such a central role in driving good governance and that's part of the reason why the UK is well ahead of many, many other countries in relation to sports governance.'

Nixon's example of how Sport England and UK Sport control the purse strings and expect good governance of the country's federations in order to qualify for funding, reminded me of the SASCOC/National Lotto Distribution Agency fiasco mentioned in Chapter Two.

It seems hard to fathom how people like Harold/Jacob Herald Adams, Hajera Kajee, Gideon Sam and Tubby Reddy would be capable of pulling the strings at places like Sport England or UK Sport the way they have managed to do in South Africa.

However, that does not mean an investigative sports reporter should take it for granted. Go and probe. There is no telling what you might uncover.

As for the American scene, Pope mentioned the country lends itself to an easy example of peculiar sports legislation since they were virtually the only country in the world where American football was played, 'Whether adults or children are playing there are various laws that govern the game and there are differences.'

Fenelon added that there were not particular laws but rather processes that he would describe as "quite Irish". He said, 'Consider the psyche of the Irish. They are quite anti-establishment. They don't mind a rule because it's rarely enforced. When I see player disciplinary issues occurring within organisations, I'm sometimes baffled by the process which really doesn't bear any resemblance to fair procedures.

'Sports governance in this jurisdiction, particularly up till a decade ago was hugely amateur. People weren't paid and they did it for the love of sport. Those with roles high up in the ranks became the *alacadoo* of their organisation, wearing the chains, putting on the ties, and really they had no skill set in which to improve all of that process.

'I'd say the last decade the thing has been modernised, professionalised and an increase on pressure on good governance from what I've seen through Sport Ireland, the sports council. Good governance is what they're obsessed about and we've had a fallout from our Olympic Council of Ireland, which was the national Olympic body.

'There was a huge controversy there with the former president of that organisation prosecuted and indeed convicted as I understand in Brazil for selling Olympic tickets in an unauthorised fashion. So that really translated to the abandonment of that organisation altogether and rebirth as the Olympic Federation of Ireland and at the heart of that is governance.

'What we're seeing now is Sport Ireland basically linking funding to delivery of governance through tangible documentation, which is constitutions, roles and responsibilities and ancillary governance documentation within the organisation.

'Do we have a specific law that's peculiar to Ireland? No. I would talk more around the landscape of sport and the law and what we're seeing is an intolerance for poor governance now.

'There's a big push as we bid to attract sports events to this country like the European football championships and other events and I think we have to create a culture that's seen from abroad to be as stable and noteworthy as our judicial system.

'That is a place of stability, of fairness and of doing things correctly. We're far from perfect but I think we're making good inroads.'

In this book's second chapter, you read about the dirty tricks played by the likes of Horst Dassler, Joao Havelange, Antonio Samaranch, Sepp Blatter and Jack Warner. While those men are now largely historical figures that does not mean that there are no villains present in the contemporary environment.

Consider Sam, Reddy, Adams et al. As pointed out, men like this tend to gravitate towards sports administration because they know they will be under significantly less scrutiny than if they were involved in traditional politics. Is part of the attraction of sports administration loosely defined or even weakly enforced law that offers them specific or additional protection?

The lines were clearly blurred within the statutes of these organisations. The FIFA scandal in the mid-2010s saw Blatter announce that the organisation needed to clean itself of a dirty image brought about by various corruption and bribery scandals coming to light. A new ethics committee was established to investigate but with a key caveat.

Blatter and his pals were granted immunity from previous misdemeanours. In other words, despite clear evidence of villainy, FIFA's bad guys basically investigated themselves, granted themselves an amnesty and then created an anti-corruption unit to investigate future crimes only.

Thankfully, no one was falling for that nonsense and it was not much longer before Blatter quit as FIFA president and received an eight-year ban from football.

Pope argued that the blurry lines meant that other elements of the law had to come into play to preserve any kind of integrity, 'You think about FIFA and what it is as an organisation and how it impacts on a community. You're looking at bribery and corruption. Those are the things that aren't related to sport.

'It doesn't say sports law on top of it but it's just the laws that are around a particular industry, so I'd think about the contracts or the litigation. You have to split it and look at this giant industry and all the things that are impacted by that and bribery and corruption.

'We've seen that here (in the U.S.) with some of the cases related to the NCAA (National Collegiate Athletic Association) athletes as well. You saw that also with the soccer community. So much has been impacted by bribery and corruption.

'There is stuff we're still getting to the bottom of, even stuff related to the Olympics. So, I think we look at it in terms of how can law stop it and look at laws that govern civil and criminal procedure in terms of being able to bring those individuals under the purview of those laws.'

It is doubtful as to whether Blatter and his FIFA cronies would agree with Nixon's assessment of the situation. 'Sports journalists have to often understand the context and understand administrators. That is particular administrators, who have been there a long time and are, as we all are to a degree, often a product of their environment.

'When you have situations whereby a governing body or an international federation is both the regulator but also the commercial rights holder, there's potentially an inherent conflict of interest there because if you're supposed to be regulating in relation to integrity matters, but those integrity matters might have a bearing on the commercial value of your sports property, therein lies an inherent tension and there's a strong argument that the integrity side is compromised.

'To a degree, it has been like that with doping and WADA and the development of the WADA code, but there's a real argument that the integrity side needs to be taken away from governing bodies and/or separate bodies set up in relation to the commercialisation of the rights surrounding tournaments and competitions.

'Because conflicts of interest lie throughout that particular framework and I think administrators who have been in positions for a long period of time probably become a product of that but also they probably become immune to, or unaware of the issues surrounding them because they are so immersed in the fabric of the particular governing body.

'That's why it's so important that senior board roles and chair roles circle and change every few years. It's vital to have a clean and fresh pair of eyes every so often to properly guide these organisations in the right way.

'These places are political environments as well. Just as politicians in government are trying to get into office and get up to things to manipulate or enhance their positions, sports politicians do the same thing,' he said.

And you thought it was only presidents who were trying to stay in office long after their term limits had expired. Point this out to your friends who thought sports journalism was a waste of time and an inferior craft to current affairs.

Fenelon observed that bribery relating to hosting events, or match fixing, or tampering with games apparatus to gain an advantage, or betting on certain games, which contradict any moral standards are integrity issues that are ultimately governed by disciplinarians within the context of sports law.

'Specifically, the national governing body for that sport has to have a robust set of rules and regulations. If there is no offence within its rules of any of those integrity issues, then it's very hard for that offence to stick and the cornered rat fights back always and that's what we have found; where the rules aren't robust enough, rules are exploited.

'In this jurisdiction, you're great for making rules but rarely following or enforcing them because of that anti-establishment Irish psyche; so in certain sports, it's not unknown for people never to accept any guilt but to fight it all the way to the courts and further.

'Are people who are on the wrong side of the law protected by sports law in any way? I think that certainly there is a bit of institutional protection around sports governing bodies and we've seen how that institutional protection in other non-sports governing bodies ultimately leads to very corrupt organisations.

'What I always advise our clients, and we act for a lot of sports governing bodies in this jurisdiction, is that it is incumbent on them to review their rules and regulations regularly and not just internally or have committee members tweak at the edges, patch or quilt the rules, but really robustly undertake a review because if they don't have a good set of rules, bad people get into power and stay in power instead of being removed.

'We've got a number of examples of controversies in Irish sport usually to do with bad governance and that bad governance usually occurs because people stay in power too long. They surround themselves with yes men and women who won't upset the apple cart and it becomes their personal fiefdom instead of serving the greater good of the sport and actually the sport suffers as a consequence.'

This also calls into question how well the average sports journalist understands laws relating to sport. While it can sometimes appear as if many sports reporters fall short in their knowledge of the law, it was not always the case, according to Nixon.

'I've come across and spoken to plenty of journalists who know their way around certain areas of law. It tends to be specialist press, or specialist industry press who might be focused on the sports betting industry. That's where their linear focus lies and the legal issues in that space are quite narrow as well, so they quickly pick up on what the core components are.'

Nixon's remarks about reporters who specialise in certain areas having a better grasp of that concept should come as no surprise. You would expect a cricket beat reporter to be well-versed in that sport in comparison to basketball for example.

The problem is that in the modern newsroom more and more it is being expected of reporters to cast their nets wider. It is not realistic to expect a reporter to be an "expert" on so many different topics. 'It's far harder for a feature writer at a broadsheet for example to have that level of granular connection to a particular industry sector and therefore, the law that is relevant to it.

'I guess there are those journalists who have less intricate knowledge but it's difficult to see how that challenge is met because journalists live in such a fast-paced environment. They're always fighting against deadlines, so finding a way to enhance that knowledge and develop skills that is going to benefit the product is very important,' Nixon pointed out.

Fenelon opined a lack of legal knowledge around sport was almost to be expected, since sports journalists by their very nature were "anoraks who love sport" rather than keen legal students. In sports-obsessed Ireland, he said, 'Most kids are reared playing six or seven sports and they whittle it down to two or three as the years go on.

'I think we have a very good calibre of sports journalists in this jurisdiction. They love their sport. They're usually ex-players themselves and have very strong links with the sport but none, if any of them, understand the legal machinations that go along with that.

'So, when you get a nice juicy story of a player disciplinary or a welfare issue, nobody really delves into how the process works. It is difficult with the column inches that they're confined to and the word count they are limited to. Then you have to ask questions like, does the readership really want that kind of content?

'Do they really want to see intricate understanding of the rules? Do they wanna see stories about possible sanctions and looking at the whole process? I think the journalists are playing to their readership and therefore, it doesn't really demonstrate a great knowledge of law.

'Would it help if they did? Well, I think people call out certain players and are maybe challenging anti-doping prosecutions better. I feel our journalists in this jurisdiction can be a little bit soft on players because they need access to those players. They want to be player-friendly to get those one-to-one interviews and they therefore aren't asking enough hard questions.

'I come back to anti-doping. Is testing widespread enough in this jurisdiction? I don't think so. Are journalists making enough noise about it? I don't think so. Why? Because they understand they have to keep the players onside. You don't become anti-player because then you're a pariah.'

Fenelon raised some important issues. Many sports reporters are wary of rocking the boat for fear of losing access. Just in the last decade, two South African cricket writers had their Cricket South Africa accreditation revoked because the regime at the time were unhappy with their reporting.

While I would not advocate for deliberately trying to have your credentials taken away or have any future accreditation applications rejected, you can rest assured that 99% of the time if the board members at a sports federation do not like you, then you are probably doing your job well.

That said access to players and coaches, as well as chairmen and other administrators, are an important element of the job but it is not impossible to do your job without access to them. Report fearlessly and without favour and make sure your sources and your facts are accurate.

What will likely happen is they will cave and grant you an interview to "clear their name" or they will issue a press release dealing with the allegations. Be on the lookout for phrases such as "We will not be making any further comment at this time" at the end of that press release.

In the event that they do not comment, directly, or indirectly, take heart that eventually they will be out of office, you will be vindicated and regain the access to that sports body. Play the long game.

Pope called a lack of legal knowledge on the part of sports journalists, one of the biggest issues facing good reporting, 'I think that's why we've been behind on a lot of different things. If something happens now, we're scrambling around trying to figure out what this means and what the impact is and I think that is a disservice to the audience if there isn't someone there making sense of it for them.

'I think that's why journalists that have a legal background, such as myself, are important to sports law and have to inform audiences on a wide range of issues that are involved. Having the depth and knowledge to be able to be a sports analyst and report on the information is so important. And all of that is before you even begin to try and tell a story.'

The reality is that a reporter is expected to regularly break stories and this often can lead to friction with those in authority. How much protection does the law give sports journalists from that point of view?

According to Fenelon, in the Republic of Ireland, 'There's the whistle-blower legislation, which is usually confined to inside an organisation that journalists don't belong to if they're breaking the story. In that regard, that doesn't really apply to them but journalists are given every protection when it comes to not having to reveal their sources.

'I think it's recognised to have a balanced democracy. Freedom of speech matters, as long as it's not offensive or hurtful and I think I have yet to see a journalist having been forced to reveal their source even in the most pressurised boardroom dramas under the commercial side of things.

'I would say that in terms of breaking the stories, journalists are always protected and they will always protect their sources and so they should continue to do so.'

In the United States, it depends on how the news comes out, while there are also whistle-blower laws Stateside, as Pope pointed out, 'Somebody being a whistle-blower is how a lot of information about corruption is found but you also have laws that protect victims that report crimes. It depends what those types of crimes are.'

In Great Britain, journalists also enjoy protection as Nixon explained, 'Provided journalists follow the rules of their own journalistic code, then there is protection. For instance, if they are going to break a story, the code will say they need to engage with the other side of that story.

'Let's say a journalist is breaking a story about something that's happened within a particular governing body, the right proper thing to do would be to reach out to the Chief Executive of that governing body and seek comment, whether it be contextual comment not for publishing or a comment for publishing.

'That's what they should do to make sure that the journalistic piece is suitably balanced. Provided they do that, they are pretty well protected because ultimately their responsibility is to hold the industry to account and particularly, senior administrators within the industry.'

It is comforting to know that there is legal protection for journalists. It is also true that sometimes journalists make mistakes and report erroneously. A typical example of this would be where somebody has been accused wrongly of doing something by the journalist, but their source was simply misleading them.

You might think it is something that only happens to inexperienced reporters, smaller media organisations and/or larger media houses that have lesser reputations but that is not necessarily the case. Even The New York Times has made errors and has had to issue apologies and corrections.

If a famous title like that commits occasional errors, be sure that you and your media house will also get it wrong eventually. It is a case of when, not if. Nevertheless, there is legal protection against these errors too.

Pope said misreporting was where the American system of protecting the free press came in. He cited the famous New York Times versus Sullivan case on defamation in terms of what papers can actually publish. It is considered a landmark decision protecting freedom of speech protections as per the First Amendment to the U.S. Constitution restricting the ability of American public officials to sue for defamation.

The United States Supreme Court unanimously ruled in favour of the newspaper. The Court said the right to publish all statements is protected under the First Amendment. The Court also said in order to prove libel, a public official must show that what was said against them was made with actual malice "that is, with knowledge that it was false or with reckless disregard for the truth".[77]

---

[77] United States Courts. (n.d.). New York Times v. Sullivan Podcast. [online] Available at: https://www.uscourts.gov/about-federal-courts/educational-resources/supreme-court-landmarks/new-york-times-v-sullivan-podcast.

Pope added, 'When publications make statements that are negligent, they still issue corrections all the time. That's something that is right out actionable but if a paper intentionally goes after someone and writes something that is defamatory, that's another story.

'A big issue is that when it comes to libel, which is written defamation, there has to be shown intent to be able to damage the individual or organisation's character. Saying, "Hey, we intend to harm this person" is a little different, so proof has to be pretty significant to be able to prove something like that.

'Mistakes with news that's breaking, and information that's not presented properly, may get someone fired in terms of liability for that publication. A reporter doesn't have to be afraid but you could lose your job but then we get into labour law and that offers protection for journalists, and there are different contracts that govern how they present their material and that nature.'

In the Republic of Ireland, it usually involves a cease and desist letter from the player or the sports organisation's legal representatives to the journalist, who then passes it on to the editor of that publication, who in turn passes it on to the legal team, who will then either recommend a retraction and an apology in the publication in the subsequent edition, or robustly defend it.

Fenelon added, 'In fairness to the press in this jurisdiction, they are under pretty strange defamation laws which they feel doesn't allow them to call out enough. I think there's some truth to that. I think that it is very easy to be defended in this jurisdiction.

'The law in terms of the defamation act, which was more recently passed in the last decade has tightened up things, under pressure probably from the press lobby, and so one must bring a defamation action against a publication within one year of the publication as opposed to within three years.

'Also, I think it's rare enough that a journalist will be personally named in the proceedings. It's usually the publication, outside of the fact the journalist has written an erroneous reference to a player or sporting body.'

Nixon reflected that while there was protection for journalists who have misreported, there is a process that has to be followed to avoid legal challenges like a court case, 'The protection they have will turn on the facts and the steps they've taken to ascertain the veracity of the story or ascertain the facts connected to the story.

'There is obviously a journalistic code over here and if a complaint is made to the press complaints commission, there is obviously an independent arbitral process that will investigate that and potentially, there could be sanctions through that process for journalists but I would imagine that provided they go about things the right way, or are seen to be going about things the right way they should be fine. The press complaints commission is active here and it will generally investigate complaints when they are made.'

As an employed staff member, labour law will inevitably become relevant. In some countries, there is more protection for full-time employees than their freelancing counterparts but the latter are not always out there alone left to fend for themselves.

Fenelon mentioned the matter of being employed full-time or on a freelance or contract basis was more significant than ever, 'If you look at the newspapers in this jurisdiction, and it's no different to what's happening globally, it's very much become an online forum and people aren't buying physical publications anymore, certainly below the age of maybe 45.

'That's really affecting matters for our sports journalists in terms of security of a job. Some operate on a freelance basis, others are on a contract basis, or full-time employees. Full-time employees really are the gilded few, and there are very few of them left.

'They are under increasing pressure from blogs, forums and sports anorak enthusiast forums. I think it's a harder place to make a living. Labour laws are no different, no matter what your profession is. It is very hard to fire someone in this jurisdiction unless you follow the correct process.

'There's usually a disciplinary process, a redundancy process and anyone who is fired and hasn't followed that process almost always follows an inevitable sanction through compensation orders to our workplace relations commission and higher up courts.'

It is good to know that it is difficult for an employer to fire someone in the Republic of Ireland but that should never be a reason for you to rest on your laurels. Things can change very quickly. Today's safety could be tomorrow's volatility, for all you know.

In Britain, the labour law is more likely to help you if you are employed whereas freelancers need to be more careful with how they go about their craft. Nixon explained, 'If they are employees, they will have all of the usual statutory protection, particularly if they have been in employment for two years' continuous service albeit in my experience a lot of journalists, and increasingly this is the case, are independent contractors.

'In many ways, that's a choice. It means, particularly feature writers, can write for whoever they want. They can go off and pursue other opportunities like write books, so it keeps them flexible but labour law is not going to protect journalists who set themselves up in that way. Labour law and employment law in the UK will only protect employees.'

As you may have noticed legal matters, whether applicable to journalism, employment or protection, differs depending on the jurisdiction and trade unions also become part of the conversation as Pope remarked, 'Journalists have labour law protection but first and foremost, you have to determine whether they have a union or not.

'Then you have collective bargaining and arbitration laws that govern those particular unions with the papers that they work with. Some of the larger organisations do have unions.

'Surprisingly, some of them may not but then if there isn't a union then you're looking at whether they are a contract employee or whether they are an at-will employee and that obviously determines the employment relationship they have and then while they're on their job you also have some of the rights and responsibilities that come with their job and whether they fall short or exceed them depending on job performance and that's just general employment law.

'And then there are also other state protections that may differ that protect employees a bit more in certain states than they do in other states.'

If you are outside of the United States, or not familiar with the term "at-will employment" it just means that an employer can terminate an employee at any time for any reason, except an illegal one, or for no reason without incurring legal liability. Likewise, an employee is free to leave a job at any time for any or no reason with no adverse legal consequences.[78]

There are countless examples all over the world where sports journalists may have handled a story better had they had improved legal knowledge. I asked Fenelon and Pope to share one example from the Republic of Ireland and the United States respectively.

Fenelon cited the Irish rugby player James Cronin's anti-doping offence where the Munster prop was given a one-month ban when in Fenelon's view, it really should have been a year. 'The rugby journalists were all about the

---

[78] www.ncsl.org. (2008). At-Will Employment-Overview. [online] Available at: https://www.ncsl.org/research/labor-and-employment/at-will-employment-overview.aspx#:~:text=At%2Dwill%20means%20that%20an

pressures a player is under and not the fact that he was a professional, had undertaken numerous seminars on anti-doping, and has to take responsibility for what he puts in his body.

'Then the Irish Anti-Doping Body did not appeal the decision, which they ought to have, because of the ridiculous leniency in the sanction. No journalist in their right mind would have written so sympathetically had they known the anti-doping rules and recent CAS case law.'

Pope feels the matter around former San Francisco 49ers quarterback Colin Kaepernick's protest against police brutality and racial inequality has not been well served, 'I think that when we start talking about missing the point legally, it's not necessarily that you've missed the bare bones of the law. When we talk about America and we talk about Colin Kaepernick, who was essentially blackballed from playing in the National Football League, and we talk about what happened in the beginning, and the impact of how a sports game changed laws, that's fine but there was no addressing Colin Kaepernick's options in terms of his grievance.

'What about the power to be able to use that kind of leverage just like the University of Missouri's football team did? They had a president there who said some things that were racially insensitive and were racist towards the students there and the players refused to play the next game unless they got him out of there.'

Pope has also not been impressed by the reporting around Kaepernick's cause ever since, "In terms of how they report on NFL players, it's just whether or not they would kneel or not kneel, whether there'll be an anthem policy or not an anthem policy, and would these guys even suit up and use their power collectively and what would that mean if they did that. This is an issue much bigger than a lockout like in 2011 and now Colin Kaepernick is a bigger figure in society in general because of the murder of George Floyd and multiple changes in the law, even down to the NFL responding to players. That to me was a big miss by the media".

To conclude the discussion, I asked each member of the panel what they would say is the number one area of improvement they'd like to see in sports journalism in their country.

Nixon says, "I think there are some incredible sports journalists in the UK and we are very blessed in that regard. I do fear because of the profile of the sports industry and this is a wider issue connected to the celebrity culture as well as the sports culture, but what I'd love to see is a reversion to more proper investigative journalism and journalism that truly gets under the skin of sport and what sport actually means; the type of feature writing that someone like Matthew Said does. Ultimately media outlets are driven through advertising revenue and obviously advertising revenue needs eyeballs and eyeballs unfortunately requires a faster form of media – click bait media – and that obviously has its place and it's not going anywhere. There are so many incredible sports journalists in the UK and you feel their skills are being diluted as a consequence of that. Maybe I'm naïve and maybe the world has just moved on and there's nowhere back from that but that's certainly what I'd love to see because there really are some incredibly skilled sports journalists in the UK but I'd query whether all of them are getting the opportunity to truly use their skills".

In a fast-paced newsroom environment where many journalists are expected to multi-task and be multi-skilled it stands to reason that there will be avenues where quality is ultimately compromised.

Fenelon opines in sports journalism vis-à-vis the law, it would be very helpful if journalists understood the legal processes, 'Be it an appeal system, hearing procedure or sanctioning and justification for sanctions. There's actually quite a lot of good stuff there. I think journalists seem to think that their journalism is confined to on-field activities but quite often, like most families, sports families are ultimately dysfunctional. I'd like to see a bit more reporting on the shortcomings or the deficits of sport which ultimately translates to grass root problems. What we've seen is the trickle-down effect to use that Reaganistic phrase, from the guys and girls who sit at the boardroom table and how they act has a massive impact on the popularity of the sport, the ability to attract sponsors, the ability to attract youth to the game and to actually deliver on the pitch in terms of results and medals. It has a massive impact and I see journalists totally ignore it because they think people aren't interested in that, and perhaps they're not, which is why you have academic lawyers who would write about this all day so I think the message I would have is "Off-field activities are as important to write about". Covid-19 presented us with the opportunity to do just that so I'm really quite sad to see that journalists were delving into the past doing hacky things like talking to old, retired players about the glory days and golden oldie football and rugby players, instead of maybe doing some investigative journalism in that space. Maybe that's not their beat. They say, "Look I'm into sport" and that goes back to why they became journalists of sport because they love the sport and they crave access and in that regard are not willing to scratch beneath the surface as perhaps they should. Our national governing body for football has had a massive haemorrhage. The CEO had to resign. There's been governmental investigations and audits into governance of the organisation. That's the very biggest organisation in our country and it's not like the journalists triggered anything.

They were simply bystanders. It was as if they were as surprised as everyone else to find out about it, and I doubt that very much, but they didn't want to rock the boat. Journalists have become part of the establishment. I think sport's greatest challenge quite frankly, is integrity. What I mean by integrity is we found that global betting syndicates are willing to infiltrate our little, when I say little it's globally significantly small, domestic soccer league. Crazy stuff. Far East betting syndicates are trying to encourage individuals to compromise themselves and their team and their communities by taking bribes and if it can happen at that level, it can happen anywhere. I'm not sure that sports journalists are talking enough about that because it's like corruption. If you go to a corrupt country, corruption is everywhere. It's endemic. It corrodes the society and it actually empties society of its talent. Corruption infiltrates every aspect of society, but sport is particularly vulnerable. Betting organisations and the sponsorship of teams is something I'm uneasy about. Nobody's calling it out and I come back to sports journalism and what their mission is, and it's not just to report what's on the pitch and be loved by everybody because you have a bit of an ego stroke. It's also about calling stuff out and consistently doing so. There is just a deficit there and it's like people are pretending it's not happening. If you look at what's happening in doping and the world of doping. We're getting into genetic doping and we're well into it. People still talk about blood doping, but we've moved on and journalists know that. I think they want to be the purveyors of happiness and drama rather than the murky dark underworld of sport.'

Finally, Pope adds he would like to see people of colour be better represented, 'I feel as if those like myself are essentially the backbone of information of how we understand sports now in the modern world. The voices of people of colour have to be elevated.

'There have to be people of colour that are elevated as experts in sports law. We're in this issue of Black Lives Matter and empowerment now, so whether it's leaders such as myself speaking, or whether it's making decisions in terms of editors' positions and also in terms of ownership as well.'

Hopefully, this chapter would have given you some insight into sports law, how it works in different countries and why it would be to your advantage to educate yourself in this area. I maintain it is unrealistic to expect any journalist to be all-knowing.

That said when you are in the workplace, do not expect any of your colleagues to go easy on you for lacking knowledge in a certain area. News editors do not have much tolerance for answers like, "I don't know". This should not deter you from pursuing your dream of becoming a sports journalist though.

Instead embrace this information and then do your best to equip yourself with as much knowledge as you can to prepare yourself for your career.

Later in this book, we shall deal with typical encounters you can expect in the newsroom and what you can do to make yourself useful and also bulletproof. I actually know a journalist who reads court judgments as a hobby.

You do not have to be that dedicated or enthusiastic about legal matters but I would encourage you to at least read up on reports by other sports reporters (or better yet news reporters specialising in court coverage) to familiarise yourself with what is going on.

If you have identified a different niche within sport; perhaps one of the examples mentioned earlier in this chapter like bribery, corruption, doping, injuries and recovery, medicine, racketeering, science, sexual abuse or technology, then go all out to become an authority on your chosen topic.

A senior person at Al Jazeera once described one of our reporters as a "policy wonk dork". That might sound like an insult to anyone outside of our industry but as a reporter, you could not wish for a higher compliment. Be a "policy wonk dork" in your chosen niche.

Chapter Eight
The Window of Opportunity, Internships, Job Shadowing and Mentorships

Before we sink our teeth into the world of internships, job shadowing and mentorships, I would like to make it very clear that in the first instance, I would highly recommend a degree from a tertiary education institution, as discussed in Chapter Six. Even though it is possible to enter journalism without a certificate, diploma or degree, it is a potentially career-limiter.

You could miss out on the opportunity to live and work in China or the United Arab Emirates for example, and some of the more elite news media houses, may very well insist on such qualifications regardless of your experience. You might say to me that you have no interest in being based in countries like China or the UAE but the truth is that no matter how well we attempt to plan our lives, there are many variables for which we simply cannot account.

You do not know what the future holds. It is better to be prepared rather than find yourself suddenly retrenched, unable to find work locally and find yourself blocked from the only opportunity you might find in that moment because you lack the qualifications.

Moreover, do not forget that China and the Middle East are areas where so much sport takes place. Imagine if you were based in China in the lead up to the 2022 Winter Olympic Games, or in Qatar ahead of the 2022 FIFA World Cup.

That said if you are unable to afford university fees then there are alternative ways into journalism and perhaps after saving up for a few years you can then complete that degree, which is more or less what I did. In fact, I had already been working in the media for 15 years before I finally graduated.

With that in mind, I think it places me favourably to explain this particular route. After all, your experiences outside of the classroom, through extracurricular activities and internships, can also equip you with sufficient knowledge, skills and tools to break into this competitive field.[79]

I want to start with internships. An internship is when a company gives candidates (sometimes specifically defined, as students for example, but not always) the opportunity to gain work experience at their establishment. Sometimes there can be some small compensation but it is not always the case.

An internship, from your point of view, is a wonderful opportunity to work in a particular job or role, gain experience, hone your skills and acquire knowledge that they usually do not teach you at university.

The first television news channel I worked at, e News Channel (now eNCA), was a great place for internships. During my time there, it felt as if the place was a conveyor belt of interns. There were always interns at e and there was a regular supply of fresh interns. This was mutually beneficial as both e and the interns were testing the waters.

From the company's point of view, if an intern showed promise, they could bring them on board as freelancers or full-time staff. In the case of the interns, if they worked hard and impressed the bosses, it was potentially the start of an exciting career in journalism for them.

The flip side was also mutually beneficial. If the intern was clearly not up to it, the company knew that they would soon be rid of them, and in the meantime could downgrade their responsibilities to mundane tasks. Similarly, from the intern's point of view, they might discover during the internship that maybe their interests lie elsewhere.

While that might come across as meaning journalism was not for them, that was not necessarily the case. For example, you might find yourself in an internship where you are working on the business desk, but your true passion lies with sport. You likely had a mediocre, or worse experience and decided that journalism was not for you.

If you are an aspiring sports journalist, make sure that you tell the company, recruitment officer, HR person or whoever the internship placement person is, otherwise you are just wasting each other's time. That said it could happen that

---

[79] Andrea Koppel (2019). How to Break Into Journalism, Even If It Wasn't Your Major. [online] Time4Coffee.
Available at: https://time4coffee.org/how-to-break-into-journalism-even-if-it-wasnt-your-major/ [Accessed 31 May 2020].

you are offered an internship and the only opportunity is away from the sports desk. Take it.

Do not hesitate and then what you can do is once you have fulfilled your duties, you can make your way to the sports desk, where you can introduce yourself and make sure they know you are interested in helping them out. Chances are that eventually this will be noticeable enough and you will be moved to the sports desk for your internship, or you may be invited back for a second internship at the sports desk.

What is key is that you recognise the opportunity. When I joined P4 as a sports anchor on the afternoon drive show, my actual ambition was to be a radio presenter. I did not really want to be the sports guy on the drive show, but by accepting that role, it ensured that I got my foot in the door.

I was in the industry and within range of people who make decisions about who the presenters will be. If I had turned that opportunity down, who knows what path my career may have taken? I would like to think that it would have worked out well anyway, but this can be a cut-throat industry.

For all I know, I might still be at Radio KC, where I had the most wonderful time, but I was not earning a salary. It is significantly easier to turn down a big radio station when you are already working at a big radio station. When you are at a small community radio station and you get an opportunity at a big radio station, it is a no-brainer. Take it.

What happened to the interns at eNCA? Many of them went on to work full-time at the channel and it would not surprise you to read that the ones who were offered full-time jobs were the ones who worked the hardest to impress.

They were not always from the richest neighbourhoods or backgrounds and oftentimes getting home at night required a friend or colleague doing them a favour with a lift home (there was no Uber in those days) but they did what needed to be done and now they reap the rewards. Be like them.

Although I never did an internship, I did volunteer for 15 months in community radio before breaking into commercial radio. An internship might come with compensation, but it is nothing to get excited about. It is the kind of money that should at least cover your travel expenses to and from the office with some spare change.

In 2004 at Radio KC, I was hosting the afternoon drive show while still hosting the Saturday late morning show. Someone with a shrewd legal and labour brain determined that I was working too many hours at the radio station and because of this, they were obliged to pay me something.

The first solution was to drop the Saturday show, which I was happy with since prime time presenters seldom host shows on weekends anyway, plus it meant my weekends would free up, which for a 21-year-old was great news. However, I was still working too many hours to legally be considered a volunteer.

The solution was to pay me a tiny salary. It was small but it did cover my petrol expenses for the month with some money to spare too, which I usually spent on a snack and a soft drink before or after my show.

Be aware though that there are many internships that do not offer any compensation. It would be better if they were renamed "volunteerships" I think but then I was probably guilty of that myself when I was the executive editor/co-owner of *The Sports Eagle*, a sports news website.

I needed writers and posted online adverts for internships. I made it crystal clear to all the interns that there was no salary on offer, but they would receive extensive experience, mentoring and the opportunity to have their work published regularly.

Moreover, they were free to leave at a minute's notice and oftentimes, I even assisted them in finding full-time employment. I loved running *The Sports Eagle* and helping so many of our writers, who tended to be students. During a two-year period, many of them had the opportunity to interview some of South Africa's top sportsmen and women, including world champions and Olympic medallists.

Some of them "graduated" from our small operation to go and work at places like eNCA (I even personally recommended one writer to my old boss) and News24 (the country's biggest news website). I was very proud to have been privileged enough to play a small part in their development.

There is power in taking an internship, voluntary or otherwise, but I need to stress once you are in, then the ball is truly in your court. The onus is on you to make a success of it. I had one writer at *The Sports Eagle* who was given a Netball World Cup match report as his first assignment on his first day with us; a Saturday morning.

All our writers worked remotely, so about 30 minutes after the match finished, I texted him to see if everything was okay. I was concerned that perhaps he did not fully understand what was expected of him. He assured me the match report was on its way.

The way it worked was that the writers would watch the matches at home (sometimes I arranged accreditation for them and they could go to the stadiums and cover matches from there, and also attend post-match press conferences) and then write a short match report before emailing it to me.

I would sub the script and then post it to the website before promoting the article via Facebook and Twitter. After two hours, the match report of this particular intern still had not arrived and after several text messages, he admitted to me that it would not be possible for him to write the piece as he was in Lesotho for a funeral!

I relieved him of his duties right there and then. Even though this guy was new, I could not believe he would pull a stunt like this on his first day with us. Who knows what else he might be capable of? Do not be like that guy. Imagine you got yourself an internship at CNN or the BBC and you let your boss down like that on Day One.

The reality is that if this guy had told me earlier in the week, or even the day before, he would be out of the country for a wake, I could have arranged for one of the other writers to take up the assignment. I would have been very understanding and suggested he rather start the following weekend, or even the weekend after that.

An internship does not have to take place at a television news channel. You could intern at your local community newspaper. The point of the internship is not to do it at the most prestigious media house, but instead to gain valuable experience.

You might think that your little local paper does not have much you can learn from but do not underestimate the power of local information and the contacts local journalists have. If riots break out in a smaller city or town, the local politicians and authorities will give interviews to the local newspaper, radio stations and television channels first because they know them.

Yes, it is true if CNN comes to town, they will get the interview anyway because they carry the weight of their reputation but the mayor or the fire chief is likely to tell the local reporters things they may not tell the bigger networks. The same applies to local players and coaches.

Working at a local publication allows you the opportunity to get to know the players and coaches from the local teams. This is especially powerful in smaller markets.

The local press that cover the Green Bay Packers often have better trust with the players, coaches and administrators than their counterparts covering the New York Giants for example. The reason is because in Green Bay, the Packers are the only team of significance, whereas in New York, the Giants are just another team and it can happen that some publications might send different reporters to their media events each week. This week, a reporter could be at the Giants but next week, he is at the Yankees, or the Rangers.

Trust is an important element in journalism. Local reporters know about trust better than anyone. I have a great relationship with many in the tennis and boxing fraternities. I can call them any time I like and get an interview but if someone else calls them, they might be told to wait until tomorrow, or later in the week and because local reporters understand that better than most, there is a lot you can learn at your local media houses.

To get an internship, you need to check your local newspaper, websites and Facebook pages to see if they are being advertised. It is also possible they are advertised on bulletin boards at universities, since it makes sense for a media house to advertise there for journalism interns.

While that is a good starting point, I would recommend you be more proactive. Pick up the phone and call every news media house in your area. You decide how far you are willing to travel. If you are in Dallas, then Seattle may be too far away.

Mind you, Wichita Falls may be too far away. Ultimately, you have to decide. When I phoned the community radio stations in Cape Town, I also called Radio KC in Paarl and MFM in Stellenbosch. Both those towns were about 30 minutes' drive from where I was living and that was doable for me.

However, I did not even bother phoning Eden FM in George, a town approximately 400 kilometres from Cape Town. You will have to determine for yourself how far is too far away.

Often a university degree or studying towards a university degree is necessary to qualify for an internship. Sometimes, you do not need any qualification and your ambition and enthusiasm can be sufficient to get in. Consider the following two examples of Spencer Bokat-Lindell and Kelly Wallace.[80]

---

[80] Andrea Koppel (2019). How to Break Into Journalism, Even If It Wasn't Your Major. [online] Time4Coffee. Available at: https://time4coffee.org/how-to-break-into-journalism-even-if-it-wasnt-your-major/.

Bokat-Lindell, at the time of writing, an Associate Editor at *Axios*, wrote for his local *Montclair Magazine* as a teenager while in high school; basically an internship. He would go on to serve as Managing Editor at Yale's *The New Journal.*

Later, he would write about his experience in the fine dining industry for Narratively.com and used that as an example of his work to gain an internship at *Harper's Magazine,* the summer after he graduated.

Wallace helped produce news and feature stories at Penn UTV, the University of Pennsylvania's campus TV station. Again, basically an internship which, believe it or not, helped her get a summer internship at the station's local NBC affiliate in New York City.

Do not underestimate the power of an internship at an affiliate network. In the United States, there are so many local television news channels and many of them are affiliated to the big networks like NBC, CNN and Fox. The next part of Kelly's story is one I really like.

She moved to Washington, DC, where she slept on a friend's couch to get closer to where she believed journalism jobs would be easier to land. Kelly finally got a break when the U.S. Chamber of Commerce hired her as a production assistant.

With a year's experience, and knowledge she gained working in production, even though not at a news organisation, Kelly was able to land an assistant producer position at CNN. And from there, she built an impressive track record as a producer and eventually, as on-air correspondent. That could be your path.

Remember that sometimes just being equipped with your journalism degree will be sufficient to get you into the job market but it is not always the case and something you might want to strongly consider while studying is an internship during your holidays or on weekends.

That way upon graduation, you have already built up experience, skills and knowledge, plus the company will know you quite well by then and would be more likely to bring you on board full-time. I know a guy who spent his weekends working at a nursery.

When he graduated from high school, the nursery offered him a full-time position as a manager. I know you are more interested in football than flora, but the principle is the same.

I also want to touch on job shadowing and mentorships. They are very similar but not quite the same thing. Let us begin with the former. Job shadowing is when you contact a company and express your interest in a specific area of work, in your case that would be sports journalism, and you ask them if you might be able to come in and shadow someone who works in that job.

All the job shadowers I have ever encountered have been teenagers still in high school, but there is no rule against anyone older engaging in job shadowing. If anything, I would encourage it to students and even adults. If you are interested in sports journalism, why not see if you can shadow a reporter, producer or presenter for example?

On a practical level, what this might entail is that on a certain day, you would report for duty at the company. You would likely meet a recruitment or HR staffer who will likely give you a short tour of the premises before introducing you to the person you will be shadowing.

I have never had anyone shadow me while working as a presenter, but I had several shadowers when I worked as a reporter. I tried my best to explain to them what exactly it was that I did on a daily basis, how I went about my craft and tried to be objective in giving them the pros and cons of the job.

Job shadowers are usually people who are specifically interested in the area of work they are shadowing, so the people I had shadowing me were always very interested in sport and television news, which was great and if you are shadowing a reporter that means you will likely have the opportunity to accompany them to interviews, press conferences and so forth, unless specific accreditation is required.

In South Africa, the environment was a little more relaxed, so I was able to take shadowers with me to watch some of our national sports teams train and then they attended the press conferences with me afterwards as well. However, there were one or two hairier moments I must share with you.

It was August 2011 and I had a new colleague. Out of respect, I will not mention his name, but he was not an actual journalist. He had no relevant qualifications; he worked at the local municipality's electricity supply call centre.

This person helped my then-boss with his electrical bill that had been erroneously inflated and since there were several back-and-forth phone calls, this guy managed to discover that my boss was the head of sport at a big television news channel. I do not know what he said or did but the next time we had a vacancy, this guy was working at e News as a sports reporter.

Talk about identifying an opportunity and moving in for the kill like a shark who sniffed blood! Which of course is exactly what I am encouraging you to do in this book.

Now even though this person was not an actual job shadower, on his first day at the office, he accompanied me to the season launch of the local football league. The Premier Soccer League (PSL) traditionally hosts a media event before the season kicks off.

The PSL chairman, sponsors, team players and coaches are all present and it is a great opportunity to conduct some interviews in a more relaxed environment, plus in those days, the PSL was legendary for the great food and snacks it provided to the media, so we all looked forward to their press events.

Nevertheless, I told my new colleague to just follow me around and observe. Imagine my horror when he told me on the way back to the office that one of the questions I asked in the press conference was actually one that he intended to ask but the media liaison picked me out instead of him.

His job that day was certainly not to ask any questions at the press conference. He was just there to observe. If you find yourself in a job shadowing situation, do not do anything that could potentially embarrass the person who you are shadowing. Be like a literal shadow; you are there but no one really notices you. Your time to ask questions to players, coaches and administrators will come.

Something else I liked to do with those who were shadowing me was give them the microphone and give them the opportunity to record a PTC, or piece to camera. A PTC is also known as a "link" at some television channels, and is the part of the story where you literally see the reporter providing you with information.

They are usually standing or sitting in a part of the stadium or office, relevant to the story. If you are doing a story about Newcastle United, then you might choose to record your PTC standing outside St James' Park, or better yet inside the stadium. PTCs are not limited to stadiums, training grounds or administrative offices though.

I have recorded PTCs on the London Eye with Westminster Abby behind me, on a bench beside the River Thames, on a construction site kitted in a hard hat, inside a butchery dressed in a butcher's uniform with a meat cleaver in hand (don't ask), in the cockpit of an aeroplane, and at the airport arrivals and departures halls, for example.

One of the best PTCs I did was while covering a snowboarding and skiing competition at the Tiffendell Ski Resort in the Eastern Cape province in South Africa. As you might know, my country is not well-known at all for its winter sports. So much so that it is fairly common for South Africa to not even send an athlete to the Winter Olympic Games.

Nevertheless, one athlete that did manage to represent the country at the Winter Olympics was Alex Heath, who became the first African to compete in all five alpine skiing disciplines; downhill, combined, slalom, giant slalom and super-G, at the 2006 Games in Turin.

I interviewed Heath at the competition at Tiffendell and was delighted when he agreed to play along for my PTC. We began the sequence with him at the top of the hill. He began skiing before approaching a hill whereupon he performed a double somersault before landing perfectly.

Heath and I then swapped clothing for the second sequence, which was a close-up of me taking off the helmet before speaking into the camera. What was incredible was that some people that watched it were impressed with my skiing skills! Never to be fooled by my shenanigans, my mother immediately sent me a text message after it first aired to tell me that she knew it was not me performing those stunts.

Before I move on to mentoring, I have to share a second job shadowing horror story from the field and this should serve as a warning to you, especially if you are reading this and you are female and/or a minor, but it remains applicable even if you are an adult too.

One of my older colleagues asked me if I would be kind enough to allow his teenage daughter to shadow me one day. I was more than happy to oblige. As I recall, his daughter was 16 years of age at the time and interested in sports journalism.

On the day that she visited our premises, I treated her exactly the same way I would any other job shadower and tried to help and advise as best I could. She was in luck, it seemed at first, as that day my assignment was to attend a training session by our national football team, followed by a press conference.

South Africa were preparing to face Niger in an Africa Cup of Nations qualifier match. One of the newer players in the squad; I shall refrain from mentioning his name to save him the embarrassment, decided that in between training drills, he would attempt to chat up the young lady shadowing me.

Unfortunately, I was busy recording my PTC at the time and missed his shenanigans. She informed me about this in the car on our way back to the office. Needless to say, I was taken aback. This player was 21-years-old at the time and in my opinion, it was wholly inappropriate for someone of his age to be looking to start a romantic relationship with a 16-year-old schoolgirl.

Moreover, where was his attention? Should he not have been concentrating on the magnificent opportunity the national team coach had bestowed upon him by calling him up to the national team? In hindsight, maybe that should have been the angle of my story for that day but I think that kind of story is perhaps better placed in a tabloid publication unless of course he had a terrible match against Niger and played a role in South Africa losing, or failing to qualify.

Ultimately, the South Africans would win that match 2-0 and my young school-going job shadower did not complain to me about any kind of harassment. That said, if you are female, regardless of age, please be aware that this kind of thing does take place and it could affect you.

There are examples of journalists finding love and even marrying players like Spain's 2010 FIFA World Cup-winning captain Iker Casillas and his reporter wife, and while I would never rule out any possibility for any person finding love, please remember that it is meant to be a professional environment.

You do not want to be a journalist accused of sleeping with players, coaches or administrators to get a story. It is unfortunate that this is an accusation that is almost exclusively one weighted in the direction of women and for that reason, if you are female, I would caution you to be doubly careful.

Do not put yourself in an uncomfortable position and if you are out in the field as a reporter and you are made to feel uncomfortable by a player, coach or administrator, there are several options available to you in terms of reporting these people for harassment.

Start by asking the person harassing you to stop. It is possible that they are unaware how uncomfortable they are making you feel. If after giving them the benefit of the doubt and they still persist after you have specifically requested them not to, then report them to their superiors and also report it to your sports editor, and if necessary your news editor or CEO.

If necessary, you can even report it to the police and do not underestimate the power of social media if your complaints fall on deaf ears. That said, please do not make Twitter your first option. That should come after you have exhausted the options I have laid out.

Finally, I want to touch on mentorships. They are similar to job shadowing but the difference is that you would look to approach a specific person with specific skills and ask them to mentor you. While job shadowing can be very effective, sometimes you could be placed with someone who might not want to help and advise you and then you get very little value.

For a mentorship, you would ask someone specifically to help and advise you. You do run the risk of being rejected; in fact, you are likely to get a few rejections. There are people who might not want to mentor you. Others might be very busy and feel they cannot commit enough time, so do not be discouraged.

My personal recommendation would be to find someone who is older and more experienced and preferably also with some spare time on their hands. I have tried my best over the years to help whoever I can, but I have to admit, it has become more and more difficult.

For example, if at the time of writing, you approached me, I would have had to politely decline to help. Why? Well, I work a full-time job, my wife has very recently given birth to our first daughter and in between working and helpingmy wife with our little baby, I am writing this book.

As you can imagine, free time was a precious commodity in this instance. Contrastingly, a colleague of mine who is in his 50s would be a better suit for you at this time. He lives in Doha, but his wife is in England and his children are all adults now.

Covid-19 restrictions had left him feeling isolated. He would welcome the opportunity to have some human interaction and no doubt, more than happy to help you. So, if you reach out to someone to mentor you and they reject your offer, please do not become despondent or hold a grudge.

They may not tell you why they cannot mentor you and in some cases, some people might just be too busy to feel they cannot give you the attention they think you require.

It is worth mentioning too that you do not necessarily need a mentor while you are trying to land your first job in sports journalism. In fact, you probably want a mentor after you have already started working. Firstly, it might make it easier to find someone to mentor you.

You could ask the most experienced reporter at your news organisation to be your mentor. Alternatively, you could take a few weeks or months to identify who you think the best journalist at the company is and ask them to be your source of advice and assistance.

One last word of advice I would supply on this topic is that if the person you would most like to have mentor you does not, or cannot help you, a great proactive approach would be for you to study this person. Observe how they work, what their habits are, and then try to emulate those as best you can.

From time to time, you can still ask this person questions related to what you have noticed and in that way, you would still receive some sort of mentoring from them without them having committed to helping you. Do not become a carbon copy of this person though but instead try to emulate their best traits and you will find that while you incorporate the best bits from their approach into your own repertoire, you will gradually begin to hone your own style.

When I first started in radio, Darren Scott was my favourite radio presenter. I was working at a community radio station in Paarl while Darren was on-air at one of the country's biggest radio stations in Durban. If you are not familiar with South African geography, I can tell you that Paarl and Durban are more than 1,500 kilometres apart, so a mentorship was virtually impossible.

However, I knew Darren's on-air skills so well from listening to him for almost all of my high school years that mimicking him was easy. For my first few radio shows, I sounded like the poor man's version of Darren Scott but then as I grew more confident I shed the "Darrenisms" and became my own person. There are still some "Darrenisms" that I use in my radio, television and even written reports sometimes.

When I started in television, I had a dilemma. It was never my intention to work in television whereas a job in radio had been my dream since before I became a teenager. When I started in radio, it was easy in terms of having a role model. I just went ahead and copied Darren Scott but I had no television presenters I looked up to.

I could not utilise the same strategy. For starters, I tried to pretend that television was radio with pictures. I treated the camera as if it were a radio mic. Further to that, I started watching what my on-air colleagues did and I gradually incorporated the skills I admired most from their repertoire into my own toolbox.

These days, I have my own style in front of the camera but in those early days when I was working out what my style was going to be, the best thing was to borrow the best bits from everyone else. That is something that you can do too but, and this might sound contradictory, the best thing you can do is be yourself in front of the camera, or behind the microphone.

If you are nervous or inexperienced, I think it would help you to have someone that you could try to emulate while you gain confidence and create your own style. Emulating those who are more experienced is a good strategy initially but after a while, you are going to have be your own person. As Oscar Wilde said, 'Be yourself. Everyone else is taken.'

Chapter Nine
What to Expect in Your First Job

In years gone by, almost all jobs were advertised in the newspapers. There might have been a few vacancies that became known through word of mouth and in some instances, aspiring candidates had to phone the companies, or even visit them in person, to enquire about possible openings. That has changed.

Today, jobs are advertised online and not even exclusively on companies' websites. There are instances where jobs have been advertised on Facebook. In fact, that is the preferred approach in some countries. And you thought completing your degree was the hard part in this whole process.

That said there are some resources that you might find useful depending on your location. In the United States, there are professional resources for journalism majors like the American Society of News Editors, Asian American Journalists Association, Native American Journalists Association, National Association of Black Journalists and Investigative Reporters & Editors, who all offer job boards, career centres, career support and the like.[81]

Take a look and see if you can find some help with these resources. If you are not an American citizen, or living in the States, try to find out if there are similar organisations where you live that might help you with job listings. The onus is ultimately on you. Do whatever it takes.

The moment you have been dreaming about since childhood is almost upon you. After years of toiling, you have graduated from university, or maybe you have completed an internship, or perhaps you have been mentored, or possibly you have passed several short courses. Whatever your path, you are about to embark on a career as a sports journalist.

---

[81] BestColleges.com. (2019). Journalism Careers | BestColleges. [online] Available at: https://www.bestcolleges.com/careers/humanities-and-social-sciences/journalism/.

After managing to successfully negotiate a job interview, you are now on the eve of taking up your first professional position as a sports reporter. You are likely filled equally with excitement and trepidation. These emotions are natural and nigh on impossible to contain.

World famous football commentator, Peter Drury advised, 'Once you've got a foot in a door somewhere that is the moment to pounce and to demonstrate first and foremost humility and a willingness to listen and to lap it up and a preparedness to do more or less anything you're asked to do. I think the worst mistake you can probably make is to walk through the door and behave as if you know it all already because you won't, and kind of build from there.'

Regardless of your pathway to this juncture, the reality is that you will be well-prepared in many areas and a rude awakening awaits in others. The aim of this chapter is to assist you in making your first few days on the job pass by as smoothly as possible, or maybe you have been in the job for a while now and find yourself struggling, in which case, this chapter might help you in terms of hitting the restart button. Nothing can prepare you for certain things, but for many circumstances, you can anticipate to a large degree.

Firstly, go over the list of equipment you might need on your first day on the job. This can be a lengthy list depending on the job that you are going to be doing. An old sports editor I worked under would often question the credibility of any reporter who did not have a pen.

There is merit in that, but it would be useless having a pen if you do not have a notepad to partner the pen; which these days is equal in might to a keyboard in its relative strength to the sword. Pen and paper are important, but in the modern environment, a smartphone can do so much more than the old pen and paper combo.

In days of yore, you had to write down information frantically. There was a technique old reporters would use called "shorthand" – a system for rapid writing that uses symbols or abbreviations for letters, words, or phrases. [82] While most Millennials have only ever heard of shorthand, and it is possible Generation Z

---

[82] Encyclopedia Britannica. (n.d.). Shorthand. [online] Available at: https://www.britannica.com/topic/shorthand.

has never heard of it, it is possible to write 225 words per minute using the technique.[83]

In the modern environment, recording devices have largely replaced pen and paper methods, so if you are not skilled in the ways of shorthand, fret not. You can simply record interviews, conversations and meetings using your smartphone. In terms of notes, every smartphone will have an app that you can use to make notes.

It is also possible that you might be expected to record video. Once again, a smartphone is your best friend. Any modern smartphone will record video that is of sufficient broadcast quality. There will be various in-house technical specifications with which your video will have to comply but those are not always related to quality and the reality is that news channels download footage off Twitter these days.

If they are happy to broadcast video that they sourced from Twitter, then there is no excuse for not using the video that was recorded on a smartphone.

The smaller the organisation you are working at, the likelier you will be expected to perform more duties. It is not uncommon that you might have to go out into the field, shoot footage, record audio and then come back to the office and edit those elements. Ask about these things in your job interview to make sure you are fully prepared.

I have worked at three television news channels and three radio stations. Two of the TV channels expected me to bring my own earphones or headphones to work. Imagine going out into the field and interviewing the president of FC Barcelona and then being unable to transcribe the interview, or cut any soundbites, because you do not have any ear phones or head phones to listen back to the raw audio.

It sounds like a very embarrassing situation and the truth is that it is the company that should be embarrassed for not providing you with the relevant equipment but do not take it for granted.

On the topic of smart phones, will you be expected to use your own or will the company provide one? None of the radio stations I worked at provided me with a phone, but I did not really need it, since I was not working as an out-and-out journalist.

---

[83] Hollier, D. (2014). How to Write 225 Words Per Minute With a Pen. [online] The Atlantic. Available at: https://www.theatlantic.com/technology/archive/2014/06/yeah-i-still-use-shorthand-and-a-smartpen/373281/ [Accessed 1 June 2020].

Even so, there were headphones; colloquially called "cans" in the radio industry, everywhere you looked and there were several recording devices that were available for the reporters to use when they went out into the field. That is how it should be.

Wherever you work, you should never be out of pocket when it comes to tools and equipment, but do not take it for granted. As you shall soon discover, there are times when you will incur costs.

One television channel I worked at provided all editorial staff with a cell phone. There was a limit to the number of minutes you could use each month for phone calls but in practice, it was very difficult to breach this limit. Unless you were constantly on the phone, it would be almost impossible to have exhausted the monthly limit.

In all the time I worked at that company, I did not once breach that limit. I did however have a SMS bundle at my own expense. I had a discount rate on 300 SMS messages per month, however, this also became less relevant as WhatsApp began to emerge in the early 2010s.

WhatsApp has made a big change in the way journalists can go about their work and now similar messaging apps like Telegram, Signal and Slack have increased the options available to us.

As bizarre as it seems, there are many people out there who will ignore a phone call or an email, but will reply to a WhatsApp message. You will have to ask a psychologist why that is the case.

If you are working on a story with a tight deadline, you will have to phone around to get comments but if your piece does not require an immediate response, why not use WhatsApp? What I have often done in the past is try the phone call first and if the person does not answer, I send them a WhatsApp message soon thereafter.

They might not phone you back, but they might reply to your WhatsApp message. I have dealt with people who seem to never answer their phone, but they will reply to a WhatsApp message almost instantly.

Not all media houses will provide you with a company telephone though. Usually, they will be happy to compensate you for the costs you incur using your own phone for work purposes. This will likely require you to keep track of your phone calls or other telephone-related expenses during the month and then submit an invoice to your employer at the end of month.

This might sound simple, but those expenses can easily get away from you. For example, if you use your own personal cell phone to make a short phone call to your local football team's media liaison and the call lasts only 30 seconds, the costs of that are minimal and it is easy to take the attitude that the administrative red tape involved in claiming that back outweighs the minimal cost, so you just go ahead and bear the expense personally.

While I have myself taken that attitude in the past, the truth is that if you make hundreds of similar short phone calls per month, the costs will eventually add up, so the onus is on you to be disciplined with keeping track of such things.

While this might sound like it could potentially become an expensive exercise, these days that is unlikely to hit your pocket too hard. At the office, there will be landline telephones that you can use to make phone calls. Some companies might block these phones and the only way to gain access is for you to use a personalised code.

That will be to help the company keep track of your expenses but as long as you can justify why you are making regular lengthy phone calls to the same number, then you will not have to worry about having any money deducted from your salary.

You are not going to have any difficulty justifying an hour a day on the phone with the national Olympic federation but your bosses are unlikely to be as understanding of you spending an hour on the phone each day with your girlfriend. That said do not feel that you are not allowed to make a short occasional personal phone call.

No boss will care if you phone your spouse to tell them that you will be staying a little later at the office than expected, but an hour a day to your girlfriend will most certainly garner a less tolerant reaction.

Other great communication tools that will not bring about a personal expense include Zoom and Microsoft Teams as well as Google Meet and Skype. While the latter two have been around for a while, especially Skype, Zoom and Microsoft Teams have really emerged strongly in recent times and boomed in popularity during the Covid-19 pandemic.

You can conduct video interviews using any of those apps at no cost outside of Wi-Fi, which most offices have now. If you are working remotely, you could try to find a Wi-Fi hotspot to use those apps and if you are forced to make a payment, keep the receipt so you can claim it back.

Once you are in a Wi-Fi zone, you can simply use a screen recording app, which comes standard with a smartphone, and then you have managed to work your way around a potential problem.

While some of these solutions might initially seem "cheap and nasty", the truth is that media coverage is evolving all the time and as mentioned earlier in this book, there are YouTube videos and channels that have more than one million views, likes and subscribers, that feature video quality that is so amateurish that it would never be played out on air at a commercial broadcaster.

This is not saying that quality is not important or that it is okay to compromise. Certainly not. Instead the point is that if you have a smartphone and someone else has the most expensive camera equipment, you can still cover the story, do it justice and deliver a story of sufficient quality that will not disappoint your audience.

Remember what Seen co-founder Yusuf Omar said about audiences never having been so forgiving of glitches. They want a quality story, so give it to them.

If you are a camera operator, the company you work for will provide you with an equipment bag that will typically consist of a camera, several alternative lenses, a tripod, a boom pole, ear or head phones, a light reflector, microphones (usually a lapel and handheld mic), extension cords and various other cables, extra batteries and a light.

There are fancier additions like drones for example, depending on the organisation you are working for. Often, a cameraman will also carry satellite equipment like a BGAN portable terminal, AviWest or Dejero to facilitate live broadcasts from the field.

If you do not know what any of those are, they are simply devices that use satellites or broadband to create a live link for broadcast purposes. Unless you are a cameraman or producer working on the technical side, you will not need to know about these products outside of recognising their names.

In terms of expenses, a camera operator will never be expected to provide any of his or her own equipment unless they are freelancers or entrepreneurs in which case your hourly or project bill will have to factor in those expenses.

It might also be the case that you are required to use your own laptop. Most companies will have desktop computers at their work stations but it is not unheard of for some staff to use their own laptops, just as they sometimes use their own smartphones, head phones and so on.

Outside of freelance or entrepreneurial activities, I have never had to use my own laptop for work purposes and this will likely apply to you too but it is best to make sure with your employer and then to check what exactly the expectations are from their side. It can also be the case that you might choose to use your own laptop.

For example, you could be on an assignment and you might use your own machine to open a Word document to write a script and then you might email that script from your personal address to your work address. It is a simple example, but these kinds of things happen all the time.

Would this example warrant claiming an expense claim? Probably not but if you are using your device for work daily, then you might want to reassess.

The next topic is the dress code. Most media houses are very casual when it comes to dress codes but it is best to make sure. Each of the radio stations I worked at people dressed as they pleased. The only exception was the retail radio station, Feel Good FM, which was based at the head office of the retail company Pep.

Even though I was in the studio presenting radio shows in a Metallica t-shirt and jeans on many occasions, those working for the company outside of its radio station sported more of a corporate look.

When I moved to television, I was told the dress code was "pretty relaxed". There was one desk producer who came to work wearing shorts, even in winter and from someone like him, all the way to the bosses who were dressed very formally, usually in a suit and tie, you would see a variety of different outfits. In most cases though, a decent shirt and a pair of jeans should be fine.

For my on-screen appearances, I was expected to don a certain look. Male reporters were expected to wear button shirts with blazers and in-studio male anchors had to wear ties to boot. I would often wear these with a pair of jeans but from time to time, I would wear a decent pair of trousers and polished shoes too.

In case, you are wondering if presenters wear a smart jacket, shirt and tie on top and shorts at the bottom, I can confirm that there are a few men who do it. Their reasoning is that if the viewer cannot see what they are wearing, then it does not matter.

One male presenter I worked with actually forgot that he was dressed this way and on his way home from work, stopped at a local supermarket to buy a few groceries. I would love to know what the astonished consumers were thinking when they witnessed this sight!

I am not aware of anything similar happening with a female news anchor, probably because women tend to be considerably more stylish than men in my opinion, but there was a female video editor who came to work one day dressed in a short black dress and high heels.

As you can imagine, she turned heads all day long. While there were no rules against what she was wearing that day, it was more appropriate for a night club than the office.

You might also want to find out about food. While that might seem strange at first, remember you are going to be spending anything from 8–12 hours at the office and in some cases, even longer than that. You are going to become hungry and need to eat.

What is the company's policy when it comes to eating at your desk for example? Many television companies ban eating at the desk. It makes sense. Can you imagine coming to work with a box of finger lickin' good fried chicken and then using your greasy fingers on the computer's keyboard or mouse? Some companies also ban drinking at your desk. Imagine spilling a soda or milkshake on the keyboard!

At the companies I have worked at, I had been banned from eating or drinking at my desk, had some restrictions, and not been banned at all, so it is best you check. It could be that the company will allow you to eat a small snack or a sandwich at your desk but not sticky ribs.

It might be that you are permitted to drink from a water bottle or flask but not a cup without a lid. One of the rules at Al Jazeera is that during the month of Ramadan, all eating and drinking at the desk is banned during daylight hours. That is because Islam is the official state religion of Qatar and its citizens are expected to observe Ramadan by fasting during the day.

Many of its residents will also fast and while it is not compulsory for residents to fast, many of whom are not Muslim, out of respect for those who are fasting, you are expected to go sit in the canteen and eat or drink there privately and out of sight of those who are fasting.

You might also want to familiarise yourself with the transport situation. I have been very blessed in my adult life to have almost always had my own car so travelling to and from the office had been quite easy but even then, what about the parking situation at the office?

Parking had been a challenge everywhere I have worked. At Pep, the situation became so challenging that eventually a couple of parking bays near the front door were designated for the Feel Good FM presenters. There were also dedicated parking bays at Heart 104.9 but they were limited, so often I would arrive for work and there would not be a free parking bay.

Thankfully, the company made alternative arrangements and an adjacent parking area was made available but even then, there was not always a bay available. In these instances, it is worth leaving your house earlier because you might need to designate 5–10 minutes just to find a place to park.

At eNCA in Cape Town, I arrived quite early in the morning, so I managed to always find a place to park. In Johannesburg, if I arrived for the early shift or on weekends, there was never a problem but parking for the later shift starting in the late morning was a nightmare.

There were simply not enough parking bays for all the staff. At one stage, some of us had to park on the rooftop parking area of a mall across the road. Soon after that, the company secured a garage about 200 metres down the road and I decided to cut my losses altogether and just went straight there instead of bothering to see if there were any bays available in the main parking area. I enjoy walking, so it was no problem for me.

The parking situation at ANN7 was disastrous. There were nowhere near enough parking bays and the company even received complaints from its neighbours because of the number of cars that were parked in the street or on curbs.

To their credit, they made an alternative plan but there was a lot of tight manoeuvring required and if you were not someone skilled at parallel or reverse parking, then you had additional challenges.

Although public transport in South Africa is not at the same level as Europe, North America or the Far East, I was forced to use trains and buses after suffering some serious car trouble. I would wake up early in the morning to cycle to the bus station in order to catch a bus to a train station.

The train would then bullet from Sandton to Midrand. Then, I hopped on another bus before I had to disembark and walk about 20 minutes to get to the office. It might sound slightly inconvenient, but I took the time on the bus and train to catch up on reading and the walk was enjoyable and refreshing plus it was a bit of exercise.

During my walks, I would often pray and think about a wide variety of things from what I might try to achieve at the office that day, to what I might buy my wife for her upcoming birthday, to wondering why I was wearing a red shirt for the third Monday in a row!

Some companies might provide staff members with transport. ANN7, for example, provided a pick-up and drop-off service for early or late-night shift staff who earned below a certain salary threshold. The wisdom was that these staff members were not in a position to afford their own cars and that public transport was either too expensive, or too difficult or even impossible to secure in the early hours of the morning or late at night.

On the topic of transport, what happens in the case of you needing to use your own car for company purposes, or if you might be required to drive a company car? There are all kinds of legal ramifications that come into play in that scenario. When I worked at eNCA, the company made a habit of employing camera operators who did not have a driver's licence.

Before I continue, I cannot emphasise enough how important it is for you to have a driver's licence in this industry. Driving to training sessions, interviews or matches are part of the job. It is essential. If you do not have a driver's licence, make obtaining one a priority. In fact, I would urge you to put this book down right now and book an appointment for your driver's licence.

Because there were so many camera operators who did not have a driver's licence, reporters were often required to drive the car to and from story assignments. In principle, I do not mind driving the car but there are a few reasons why the camera operator should drive, especially on the way back from the story.

The drive back should give the reporter time in the passenger seat or back seat to write down their thoughts on the story and the interview and if possible, even produce a skeleton script for the story that will be put out on air later. That is impossible to do if you are driving, which requires high levels of concentration.

While I could still live with that challenge, I had a genuine concern that no one in management ostensibly shared. Suppose a reporter is driving the car and is involved in a car accident. It is possible the reporter suffers some serious injuries and is unable to continue driving.

The unlicensed camera operator is then unable to take the wheel and drive to the nearest hospital. I know that there is a good chance that emergency services will appear on the scene in a relatively short space of time but there is also the possibility that with time not being a luxury, the reporter could suffer heavy bleeding, slip into a coma or the worst could even happen.

It might have been preventable if the other person in the car had a driver's licence. If the roles were reversed, the reporter could assist the camera operator onto the backseat of the car before taking the wheel and getting to the nearest hospital.

Thank God this scenario never played out during any of my assignments, but life is uncertain, and this was something that had likely already happened to someone else and similarly likely to happen again in the future.

I do not blame the camera operators who do not have driver's licences, but media companies should insist on people who are going to be going out into the field on assignments having driver's licences and quite frankly, if they go ahead and employ unlicensed drivers, they should partner with a local licencing department to facilitate the process for their unlicensed employees. It is in everyone's interest.

Interestingly, the camera operators I worked with were all required to sign an insurance document to protect themselves, the company and the company car in case of an accident. I often drove cars at two television channels because the cameraman did not have a driver's licence but I was never asked to sign anything. I wonder what would have happened if I had been involved in an accident.

The other matter that you will encounter when using a company car is parking, and the expense of paying for parking. These days, there are very few commercial parking lots that can be entered without paying either an hourly rate or a flat rate.

As a sports reporter, I was often assigned to the airport to cover arriving or departing athletes and teams. If you have ever parked at an airport, you will know they do not play games with their parking fees.

Most companies are aware of these things and will gladly reimburse you for your parking expenses but that is not always the case. While working as a sports reporter at eNCA, I was invited by the Toyota Dakar Rally team to cover their testing session in the Namib Desert for a few days.

The company had no problem with me covering this story as the sponsors were paying for the journalists to go along. The arrangement was as follows: I would arrive at the office early in the morning where I would meet my cameraman, Thamsanqa.

If you are unfamiliar with the pronunciations of the Nguni languages, I challenge you to get your tongue around his name. The two of us would meet one of the company's drivers there and he would drive us to the airport. Sounds like a good, solid plan, right? Think again.

The driver was not there at the appointed time. We waited a few minutes before I became uncomfortable and so I called him. There was no answer. After the third attempt at calling him, he eventually answered. He sounded every bit like the man who had just been woken up at four in the morning by a phone call.

After he estimated how long it would take him to dress himself and drive to the office, I determined that it would put us under too much pressure, and we ran the risk of missing our flight.

I took the decision to use my own car to drive Thamsanqa and me to OR Tambo International Airport. I would pay for the parking expenses myself and then claim it back when we returned from Namibia. We arrived at the airport in time to have our passports stamped and follow all the other procedures that international travelling involves.

In my opinion, we produced some really good work from the Namib Desert. I was very proud of our efforts and we had a lot of fun during our down time. The organisers were kind enough to take us for a desert dune bashing session, we were able to join a rally driver in a car for a "hot lap" and we were treated to some really good food.

After a few days, we were back in Johannesburg and the parking expense amounted to R450, which at the time was approximately $53. That is quite a large unbudgeted expense for an overworked, underpaid sports reporter. Nevertheless, I intended to just claim it back when I returned to the office. I filled in the relevant forms and submitted my claim.

Our head of news called our head of sport in to discuss this expense. My line manager told me the boss looked at the paper and told him bluntly that this expense was not going to be reimbursed. The boss's argument was that a driver had been allocated to the story, so there was no need for me to have used my own car and my own money.

The fact that the driver had overslept and that my being proactive saved the story was seemingly not a factor. If I had not used my own car, the chances were high that we would have arrived at the airport too late and missed our flight. The sponsors and organisers who were paying for us to accompany them to Namibia would have wasted their money and it would have damaged our relationship and reputation with them for future assignments.

Apparently, that was not important and suddenly my line manager was left with this bill. I felt awful. I could see that he felt bad about it too. He supported what I had done but now he was somehow in the red. We reached an agreement to split the expense but neither of us should have been R225 worse off anyway.

About eight months later, I was again invited by the Toyota Dakar team to join them for testing in Namibia. I wonder if that invitation would have been extended if we had failed to show up at the airport on the previous occasion.

Before we finish this chapter, there are a few other things to be mindful of on your first day at the office. Even though you might have acquired a lot of knowledge before landing this job, there are many practical elements you are not well-versed in.

Be mindful of that. Nobody likes a know-it-all and especially not the new guy who sees himself as the authority and is taking it upon himself to lecture and advise people many years or even decades more experienced than he.

Be humble. It will serve you well in your early days at the office and do not assume that you are good at your job. Approach each task with enthusiasm and the attitude that it is an opportunity for you to prove your worth to your new colleagues, line manager and other bosses. Your value will shine through soon enough.

It might even happen that after a while you realise that you are the star performer on the team. This happened to me at Radio KC and again at ANN7. In the case of the former, I was a starry-eyed young upstart just thrilled to be working in radio.

I have already shared with you the disaster that was my first 10 minutes on radio but after that, I settled and became more comfortable. That was on Saturday, 20 March 2004. About two months later, it was obvious to everyone at the radio station, including myself, that I was one of their best presenters.

It made me feel good of course but I was not resting on my laurels. I knew I had to continue to improve not only to maintain that status, not only in the hope of becoming the very best presenter at the radio station, but to become so good that I could land a job in commercial radio.

At ANN7, I was one of the older sports journalists on a very young team, so many of the guys would look up to me as a role model and ask for advice and mentoring. While it was my pleasure to help wherever I could, the reality is that I myself was just 30-years-old and still had much to learn.

The company employed a strategy of hiring young, attractive female models to read the news to attract more male viewers, with disastrous consequences. Many of the models were clueless about current affairs. The theory that they just had to read the script off the autocue had giant holes punched into it when supposedly difficult names needed to be read and the ladies were badly exposed.

My sports news reading impressed so much that it was not long before I was asked to take the hot seat and present the news as well. I stood in as a prime time news host on several occasions and admittedly thoroughly enjoyed it. As a little boy, my passion for sport was only rivalled by my keen interest in politics.

There was only really one experienced news anchor at the channel, Chantal Rutter-Dros; an extremely competent news journalist who had added great value wherever she has worked. After she resigned, I was asked to temporarily fill her role and for a while, I was in contention to permanently replace her.

It was very obvious during that time to me that I was highly thought of and probably the best news anchor at the channel. Granted, the overall standard was not very high, but it was a source of pride. At the same time, I had to make sure that I continued to work hard, so I could improve. If I did not work hard at improving my skills, I would never have reached the standard required to work at Al Jazeera.

It is worth adding that some of the models ANN7 employed eventually flourished. To their credit, they identified an opportunity for themselves and worked hard at improving their knowledge and skills. Some of them grew to become very competent news presenters and have even gone on to work at other news channels.

Needless to say, those who did not take it seriously and viewed it as a stepping stone to something else, failed dismally and embarrassed themselves and the channel. The reality is that no one should be looking to use a news channel as a stepping stone in television. If your goal is to one day host *Britain's Got Talent*, a news channel is not what you should consider a breeding ground.

Craig Norenbergs, former head of sport at Sky News Australia, Australian Broadcasting Corporation Radio and Sky Sport in New Zealand, has encountered many youngsters who have had their eye on the glamour job when first starting out.

He advises against announcing those lofty ambitions on your first day in the office. Instead, Norenbergs recommends keeping an open mind and learning all the different aspects of the job, 'Do not say to me on Day One, "I want to be a presenter. I want to have my own show. I want to be the face of the network". I get this a lot.

'I want to see someone who wants to get stuck in, who wants to learn the whole gamut of building a rundown. I can remember so many young people when I was a producer. I'd sit them down and I'd ask what they want to do, and they'd say, "I want to do what he does", and they'd point to the presenter's office. I'd ask, "Don't you want to do what I do? I build something out of nothing, and every day is an adventure". They'd just go, "No. I want what he does".'

Norenbergs recommends getting on with things without too much fuss when you first arrive at your new job, 'If the boss says to you, "What do you want to do?" Just say, "I want to do what you do. I want to be the boss one day."'

In fact, the big boss at Sky New Zealand and I were talking about a young guy who works with me and I said, "He's so good. One day he's going to have your job", and he said, "Great. That's what I want to hear. That's the kind of person we want working here, who maybe not tomorrow, but in 20 years, the aim is to be that person".

'The other bit of advice is to keep your head down and not upset anyone. There's a good management book called *The No Asshole Rule: Building a Civilized Workplace and Surviving One That Isn't*. It advises that if somebody is an arsehole, get rid of them. Don't work with that person.

'They're not worth it for the team and they use sport as an analogy – it doesn't matter how good the quarterback is, if they're bad for the team, just get rid of them because they're cancerous and you're better off with a better team than just having one star who everybody tiptoes around.'

As ESPN Cricinfo editor-in-chief Sambit Bal said, 'We hire people who enjoy coming to work. One of the things we tell them is that what we do here is cricket. So be true to the way, be true to cricket. I just believe that skills can be learnt but attitude takes a long time to evolve. Have the right attitude, come to work every day and enjoy your job. We are blessed to be sports journalists.'

Bear in mind that no matter how helpful you try to be or how friendly and respectful you are towards your colleagues and superiors, not everyone will like you or value what you bring to the table. This can make for a clash of personalities and some serious arguments.

Try to avoid such things, especially early on. The television industry, like most, is filled with great people as well as jerks. You will encounter both every day of your career from the first day to the day of your retirement.

A thick skin is helpful as well as the ability to identify your own strengths and weaknesses, so you can appraise yourself regularly. If a colleague, line manager or boss does not like you for no good reason that is ultimately their problem, not yours. There are more important things for you to concern yourself with.

Finally, if there is one easy thing that you can do, it is to arrive on time. There are circumstances that are beyond our control sometimes but 99% of the time, there is no excuse for not arriving on time for work. Remember you might take a while to find your feet at the office at first.

Your competence might be called into question by your colleagues and superiors in the first few weeks or even months. Do not let late coming be something they can hold against you. That is an easy box to tick and further to that be friendly, humble and show enthusiasm for tasks even if you lack the knowledge and skills in that moment.

It is an opportunity to learn and of course, always try to be helpful. People who are not yet at the required level expected of them at the office, but exhibit these traits, will almost always enjoy more leniency and patience as well as assistance, and then a few weeks or months down the line, you will see for yourself just how much you have grown, and your colleagues will notice too.

Chapter Ten
Dealing with Difficult Editors

Whether you are a veteran reporter or just starting out, the experience of working for a demanding editor is one that cannot be too far away. Sometimes, it could just be your editor pushing you to be the best that you can be. In other cases, he or she might just be a difficult individual.

Either way, you are going to have to navigate your way through this and in some instances, you might have to manage the relationship. Almost every assignment you undertake will involve a discussion with your editor, so a good relationship, or at least understanding, is important.

Your job is to grasp what your editor expects of you and to deliver on that, and where possible, exceed that expectation. Typically, your editor will assign you to a particular story for the day, or a day in the future. You will receive your instructions and then you will set about carrying them out.

One way to surely impress your editor is to be more proactive than that. You can instead propose your own story ideas. This works like a charm, particularly on "slow news days".

When I worked at eNCA as a sports reporter, I made it my business to have my own sports story ideas each day. Most television news channels are what is known as a non-rights holder, and it can sometimes be difficult to gain access to the players and coaches from the biggest teams because of various restrictions.

Their media relations tend to be tightly controlled and there is an obvious bias in favour of their media rights holders. Instead of fighting that battle, I chose instead to make a niche for myself in the sports of boxing and tennis; sports in South Africa that cry out for exposure.

Make no mistake, if one of the big teams were having a press conference, I would still be expected to attend, but on a day when our sports editor was asking us what we had up our sleeves, I always had a boxing or tennis story to pitch. As a result, I built up very good relationships with many fighters ranging from young up-and-comers to world champions, trainers and promoters. I knew that I could phone them and ask for an interview at a minute's notice in most cases.

One of the first sports editors I worked under, Edwin Kgaswe, once told me that if he had "ten Peter Stemmets and Zayn Nabbis" he could accomplish anything! Zayn was a sports reporter at eNCA at the same time I was there. We covered the 2010 Laureus World Sports Awards in Abu Dhabi together before he left to become a producer at CNN in London, where he is still doing great work at the time of writing.

He is also a good friend. That wonderful compliment from Edwin, is exactly the kind of impression you want your editor to have of you but beware because not all editors are created equal.

Edwin and I had a wonderful relationship. If he had asked me to climb Kilimanjaro, I would not have hesitated to do it. He was always encouraging, supportive and ready with a word of advice on how to do a better job next time.

However, for every Edwin Kgaswe, you might find someone with a very different approach. Another person I worked for would routinely try to rattle their staff by putting them under unnecessary pressure. Let us call this individual Nasir Hussain (obviously not their real name).

Hussain once instructed the sports department to no longer attend press conferences. His logic was that he wanted his channel's sports coverage to be different and since all media houses attend press conferences, he did not want us to do that.

Two days later, Nasir complained that the coach of his favourite local team was on two other news channels but not his own. He demanded to know why. The reason? Those channels were at the press conference that he instructed us not to attend.

This is the same person who once told me with a very proud look in his eyes, 'I love to get under people's skin because that's how you get the best out of people.' Personally, I strongly disagree. I do not believe people perform better when they are put under pressure, nor do they respond well to criticism and insults.

As a former colleague of mine once remarked about a similarly difficult sports editor, 'More sugar and less salt please.'

The sports editor will have different titles depending on where you are working. For the purposes of this chapter, the universally understood term "editor" will be used but depending on where you work, the title could range from programme editor to head of sport, manager or executive producer.

They are not always exactly the same thing, but I personally like "head of sport" as no matter what their title, that is what they are. The amount of power they possess is often limited within news organisations as sport is usually just a department within the organisation, or sometimes a sub-department.

Bear that in mind if you want to begin complaining that your editor is "holding you back", you might find someone far higher up on the company organogram is the person you need to be discussing your career prospects with instead.

If I include all the various job titles as well as temporary positions, I have to date worked under 13 different editors and they all had different personalities and approaches. I had great relationships with some of them, strained relationships with others and indifferent relationships with one or two, but what I will say is that the editors who encouraged, supported, mentored and advised staff have been the best ones.

Speaking from my own perspective, I would feel absolutely awful if I let them down in any way, whereas those who are considerably more critical would bring about an attitude almost of apathy. The truth is that if you are going to criticise and insult your staff at every turn, it quickly loses its effect and will be met with a shrug of the shoulders.

Put a different way, if I know there is no pleasing you, then I am not at all surprised when you announce how unhappy you are with my work. Moreover, I know that no matter what I do, you will be unimpressed, so now I am almost in a position where I do not care as much.

That is not a space you want to occupy but we are all human. It can and does happen. Perhaps one day, you will rise to the ranks of sports editor, or even head of the media house you are working for. Remember what you have read here. There is a time and place to reprimand your staff, but you do not want to be the person who zeroes in on the minutest of mistakes. More sugar and less salt!

Before we delve more into personality-types, I want to share a story with you from 2012 when I was assigned to cover the Olympic Games in London. A few months before the Games, we had an editorial meeting to discuss our coverage. The head of news did not attend but instead the deputy head of news attended.

The meeting seemed to be quite fruitful and then after about 30 minutes without having engaged until that moment, the deputy head of news broke his silence in a stern, assertive manner. He looked at me and barked, 'And what about the Rugby Sevens?'

I calmly replied, 'That's only happening in Rio in 2016.'

His response was a frustrated, 'Oh,' and the meeting continued.

You would have forgiven me for thinking this man only attended the meeting to look for a gap where he could attack someone unnecessarily. After the Olympics, the head of news wrote an email to all those concerned with Games coverage saying he was unhappy with the work we did.

My cameraman and I had worked very hard in London. We were up early every morning shooting B-roll, interviewing athletes, fans and administrators, shooting PTCs in fun locations and producing at least two packages a day outside of live crossings and other ancillary bits.

We would often get back to the hotel late at night and not sleep much, before repeating the cycle the next day. We both looked back at our work after the Olympics with a degree of pride and satisfaction. We knew there was not much more we could have done, especially as a non-rights holding, two-man team from South Africa.

To have a go at us like that was uncalled for, but it also proves the point I was making earlier. No matter what you do, some people will never be satisfied. This man falls into that category and I knew it then already, so his criticism, while upsetting to a degree, was mostly met with a shrug of the shoulders from me. By the way, if he was so interested in our coverage of the Olympic Games, how come he skipped our pre-Games meeting?

Craig Norenbergs has worked as the head of sport at Sky News Australia, the Australian Broadcasting Corporation Radio and Sky Sport in New Zealand. He recommends being prepared for difficult encounters, 'Unfortunately, television or any form of broadcasting, is full of those people. You will face your nemesis at some stage in your career. There are nemesis out there. The person who will make your life hell. You've got to learn now how to deal with those people because your nemesis is out there.'

Best we learn then, hey?

Earlier in this book, I shared with you the *Flag Page* theory. Larry Bilotta developed the *Flag* in 1993 after closely examining personality tests such as the

Myer-Brigg Type Indicator, True Colours, DISC as well as the Hippocrates personality rating of Sanguine, Choleric, Melancholy and Phlegmatic.[84]

The flag page theory categorises people into four distinct personality temperaments: Control, Fun, Perfect and Peace. They are referred to as "countries" and hence depending on what "country" you are from, that would be your "nationality". These "countries" are very different from one another. They have different customs, traditions, and ways of doing things, and words and even phrases that can have very different meanings.[85]

Everyone will have a primary "nationality", or home country, as well as a lesser second "nationality", or adopted country. For example, I hail from "Peace Country", while "Fun Country" is my second "nationality". My wife is a "Perfect Country's" citizen, with a second "nationality" from "Control Country".

We took the *Flag Page* test while we were still dating, and it has helped us better understand one another. For example, when my wife is fretting over a photo frame that is hanging skew by an almost unnoticeable angle, I would not be bothered but understanding that "Perfect Country" is her home country, helps me recognise that she is just being herself.

Similarly, when I start cracking "Dad jokes", she just rolls her eyes. She knows my second citizenship is in "Fun Country". I cannot even help myself, let alone stop. You can see from this very simple example that people from different "countries" see and experience things differently.

This also applies to the newsroom where there is a large variety of people with different backgrounds. You might say to me that your local newsroom is nowhere near as diverse as an international newsroom like Al Jazeera for example.

Perhaps, but if you look hard enough you will find that even a local community newspaper will have men, women, people of different religions, races, and even political persuasions. Diversity is great because it brings different perspectives to the table which makes for better discussions.

And even if everyone in your office is from the same demographic group, I can assure you that a variety of different "countries" will be represented.

---

[84] Gungor, M. (2017). Discovering your heart with the Flag Page: a simple and powerful way to truly understand yourself and others. Laugh Your Way America! Llc. P17

[85] Gungor, M. (2017). Discovering your heart with the Flag Page: a simple and powerful way to truly understand yourself and others. Laugh Your Way America! Llc. P19

Let us look at what the *Flag Page* theory says about the various home country/adopted country combinations.

Control/Fun or Fun/Control: The world's greatest leaders. They have fun, but they still get things done, and people like to follow them.

Fun/Peace or Peace/Fun (this is the category I am part of): The world's most lovable people (Thank you!). These people love to have fun and are able to easily get along with everyone.

Peace/Perfect or Perfect/Peace (the largest group): The world's greatest workers.

They get along well with others but are careful to get things right.

Control/Peace or Peace/Control: The world's best owners/managers. They get things done but are careful of the feelings of others. This allows them to communicate well on a personal level while still keeping their "eye on the ball" of what needs to be accomplished.

Perfect/Control or Control/Perfect (the smallest group): They are considered the world's strongest willed people. You better get it done and get it done right. These are the people who would be the happiest if they owned their own island country and had themselves installed as the ruling dictator.

If you work for an editor from Perfect/Control or Control/Perfect, you might want to buckle up for a rough ride. One editor I worked under was a classic example of this personality type. We shall call her Emma Hunter (not her real name).

I remember one incident where I was called out for something. Emma used the words "epic fail" to describe what I had done wrong, except of course the "epic fail" being referred to was not actually my assignment. It was the work of one of my colleagues, but Hunter saw fit to insult me in front of my co-workers. Was there an apology? Of course not. Remember what I told you previously about having a thick skin in this industry?

Finally, we have the Fun/Perfect or Perfect/Fun people: The world's best entertainers or creative people. A unique combination that is a conflicted one. In comparison to the other combinations, this one is most at war with itself. This is because Fun does not like Perfect and Perfect does not really care for Fun.[86] As

---

[86] Gungor, M. (2017). Discovering your heart with the Flag Page: a simple and powerful way to truly understand yourself and others. Laugh Your Way America! Llc. P21-22

I write this, I am thinking I might have to write a book about how Fun and Perfect are able to have a happy marriage.

The next thing I want to show you are words and phrases that people from the respective countries typically love to use and hear:

Control Country

- Grasp.
- Control.
- Get it done.
- Appreciate.
- Accomplish.
- Achieve.

Fun Country

- Really.
- Happy.
- Good time.
- Funny.
- Great.
- Fun.

Peace Country (My Primary "Country")

- No hassle (I love harmony).
- Easy way (Why must things be difficult, right?)
- Relax (Yes, please).
- Low maintenance (That's what I'm all about).
- Respect (I touched on this in an earlier chapter, remember?)
- Smart (Of course I am!)

Perfect Country

- Ideal.
- Sensitive.
- Right.
- Feel.
- Details.
- Perfect.

I hope you are starting to see certain patterns emerging. A lot of this makes so much sense and you have likely already seen it in action in your life without realising what was going on at an emotional or psychological level.

No matter what "country" you are from, you will have certain traits that make you an asset to any organisation. Here is a brief list of the attributes that are typical of the various "nationalities" when they are at their best.

Control Country

- Born leader.
- Tons of confidence.
- Goal setter.
- Independent.
- Moves quick to action.
- Bold.

Fun Country

- Enthusiastic.
- Optimistic.
- Inspirational.
- Great sense of humour.
- Loves people.
- Sincere at heart.

Peace Country

- Competent.
- Consistent.
- Witty.
- Patient.
- Peaceful.
- Good listener (Mrs Stemmet might dispute this!)

I actually ran this by my wife during the writing process and she asked if the next point is "Very good at finding things that are right in front of them?" Even though she is not from "Fun Country", my wife certainly does have a wicked sense of humour.

Perfect Country

- Faithful.
- Persistent.
- Idealistic.
- Creative.
- Organised.
- Thoughtful.

If you rise the ranks and become the editor, you might want to be mindful of the different personality traits that are typical of the different "nationalities". It will not only help you better understand the way your team members see the world, but will also help you get the best out of them.

When someone is at their best, regardless of their "country", it brings about great results. Similarly, when they are their worst, it can be a disaster for all concerned. Now no one is perfect, even folks from "Perfect Country", and so here is a quick summary to give you an idea of what attributes the various "nationalities" display when they are at their worst.

Control Country

- Bossy
- Impatient
- Quick tempered
- Demanding
- Know it all
- Arrogant

Fun Country (My Second "country")

- Talks too much (If you can't say it in 500 words minimum, then what's the point, right?)
- Exaggerates (I would never do that!)
- Seems phony (Just like Jennifer Lopez, I'm real!)
- Forgets responsibility (My wife might be able to elaborate here because I cannot think of a single example!)
- No discipline (What?)
- Easily distracted (Oh look, a bunny!)

Peace Country

- Fearful and worried
- Can't make decisions
- Too shy (Thanks to my adopted country this is not really the case but as a young boy I was painfully shy.)
- Little self-motivation
- Resents being pushed (Resents!)
- Resists change (If it ain't broke, why fix it, right?)

Perfect Country

- Remember negatives

- Moody
- Feels guilty
- Too much time planning.
- Standards too high.
- Insecure around people.
- Depressed

It might sound contradictory but "Control Country" citizens' greatest need is to be appreciated. Despite their impatient tone, inability to listen and their intense nature filled with quick words, and abrupt, to the point approach, there is a need to be appreciated.

"Fun Country" folks love being around people and see the humour in everything. They are very chatty and love having fun. Their greatest need is approval for the way they act. Have you ever seen people tell a joke and then look around the room hoping someone will join them in a burst of laughter?

You can see the anticipation in their widening eyes. I only describe this behaviour so well because I have done it myself. But only once.

"Peace Country" residents are all about getting along. Their greatest need is to gain respect for who they are, no questions asked. They are calm and productive and like to just get on with things, with little to no drama preferably.

"Perfect People" want to get it right, but they have a lot more sensitivity to their feelings. They love closely examining the details of their life and worry about things not being right while enjoying lots of little details.[87]

Now that you have a better understanding of the different personality types, I am sure you have already identified your own type. While this is very useful, I would strongly encourage you not to use your weakness, or even your strengths, as excuses for being incapable of performing certain tasks.

Work on those weaknesses. Just because you are a chatty "Fun Country" person does not mean that you cannot turn down the volume, hit the pause button and listen to what the other people in the room have to say. It might not come naturally to you, but it is not impossible.

---

[87] Gungor, M. (2017). Discovering your heart with the Flag Page: a simple and powerful way to truly understand yourself and others. Laugh Your Way America! Llc. P27-44

By working on your weaknesses and showing improvement in those areas, you will become a better individual and as a result, a better journalist too.

I would strongly encourage you to get yourself a copy of *Discovering Your Heart with the Flag Page* by Mark Gungor. Here I am summarising parts to give you an idea of what has helped me personally and professionally but nothing can substitute for reading the book yourself and then also heading over to www.flagpage.com and taking the test to determine your own "nationalities". Once you have done this and you better understand yourself, you will also begin to better understand others.

I have reached a point in my life where whenever I interact with people, I try to determine which "countries" they are from. Of course, it is a guess since I am not actually making them take the *Flag Page* test, but once you understand how the *Flag Page* theory works, you will probably be able to identify which "country" most people are from at least 80% of the time and by knowing where they are from, or more or less where they are from, you will be better equipped to deal with them.

For example, at a channel I once worked at the news editor (we are going to call him Ajit Singh) was clearly from "Control Country". Ajit loved coming to the sports desk to bark orders in an unnecessarily aggressive manner. After a while, I determined that while Singh was clearly from "Control Country", his adopted country was not "Perfect Country".

This helped me to understand that he was not interested in whether or not we actually did what was commanded, but it was more important to him that he came to us and acted in a bossy, impatient and demanding fashion to exert his authority.

Many of my colleagues were very uncomfortable with this behaviour but after I explained to them that Ajit was not interested in whether or not we actually did what was ordered, or to what degree it was done, but rather simply that the orders had been issued, they saw what was going on and began to calm down.

For the record, we did not ignore the instructions. We did carry them out as that is what a subordinate should do but there was no need to feel angry or offended. Just brush the behaviour off as Singh not being able to control his emotions. I realise that this can come across as an attitude of apathy and I would never encourage that.

Instead, it is just a way of better understanding people and equipping yourself to better deal with potentially difficult scenarios. As the old saying goes, you do not have to attend every argument you are invited to. Some battles are not worth fighting. Choose your battles.

Being shouted at to get a story on air that you are already working on, or that is already on air (yes, that has happened several times in my career because there are bosses out there who ostensibly do not watch their own channels), is something I am not interested in arguing over.

I calmly point out that we are working on it, or that it is already on air. In my opinion, life is too short to involve yourself in spats over nonsense.

IRONMAN worldwide announcer Paul Kaye has worked on-air as a radio presenter and also spent time in management, first as a programme manager and then as a station manager. He says that some managers are difficult while others actually have a method to their madness.

'That could be a brilliant manager who knows you're being lazy or it's a lazy manager who doesn't actually understand the medium and doesn't understand how to manage you and is just being very vague. I'm a bit of a petrol head. I love cars.

'BBC Top Gear for decades has been one of my favourite motoring programmes and I love to read British Car magazine and British Top Gear. When the three boys left Top Gear; Jeremy Clarkson, Richard Hammond and James May, and started the Grand Tour, I was super excited.

'I thought these guys were going to be unleashed, they were going to be awesome. I was so disappointed at first and I found some of their programmes, for me, were hit and miss, because it came across to me that they had become three old men sharing an inside joke the whole time and ticking off their bucket list at my expense because I'm paying the Amazon fee to watch them and Amazon was just giving them bucket loads of money and very little creative management.

'Whereas at Top Gear at BBC, which can be extremely politically correct, BBC had strict editorial guidelines and really forced these guys to be uber creative to get away with just a little bit of what they wanted to get away with and this made for amazing programming because they had to walk such a fine line whereas with the Grand Tour they were walking a brick wall, a very big dam brick wall. They could do anything they wanted to get away with. I felt that that was making them lazy. Management is critical.'

'The purpose of that advice is for you to not automatically assume victim status when confronted by a difficult or moody manager. That said there are

192

many out there with an axe to grind as Kaye warns, "The other problem with management often in this industry is these are people who wanted to do what you and I do, but didn't quite crack it and then they get into management and then they actually get jealous of you because you're the one with the photograph and the by-line or you're the one in front of the camera, or you're the one making more money than them."

'Not many managers can cope with their talent or their staff making more money than them, so that's another thing where as a talent, if you have ambition to go somewhere, look very carefully at the rungs of the ladder you want to climb, and against which wall that ladder is placed. Don't be weak and go into a weak environment.

'Be strong and go into a strong environment. Work with good people and try and find yourself a good manager that allows you to manage them, as much as they'll manage you because that way there'll be more of a sharing of skills and you'll get more honest feedback which will help you be a better talent.'

Craig Norenbergs' philosophy is to use each experience as an opportunity to learn, 'I don't believe in yelling or screaming. If you're a boss, trust is a very big thing. You trust them to do the job. You trust them when you're not in the office. Once, at one of those management get-togethers, they had a guy who had come across from Israel and he was an expert in negotiations.

'The advice that he gave was around the word "appreciation". For any manager, particularly in media, to be able to say to someone, "You know I really appreciate the effort that you put in there. I really appreciate the extra yard you went", is important.

'He was doing that to stop wars in the Middle East and he said in a work setting if you say to someone, "I really appreciate that" and you're a boss, it will make up for any money shortfall or any kind of angst that they've got because you said, "You know what, I can put myself in your shoes and I appreciate what you've done". It's always stuck with me that the word "appreciate" is a word that is hardly used but should be used more.'

Norenbergs conceded he had not always been able to get everything right, 'I'd like to think I learnt from every single good or bad experience. The philosophy should be, "Thank you for the lesson". You'll walk away knowing you learnt something. You might not know what you learnt but you learnt something.'

While Norenbergs is talking specifically about himself, that is a lesson that can be taken on board for anyone working in any position.

Even though this chapter is primarily intended to help you prepare yourself to deal with difficult managers in the newsroom, I wanted to include Kaye and Norenbergs to make it clear that there are managers out there who see things in a different way. Once you have worked under a difficult personality, you will be even more appreciative of a manager who knows how to help you grow.

It is worth noting that you are unlikely to need this information solely for dealing with your superiors. In many cases, this information will prove more than handy in your personal life, as it has helped my wife and I, but also when dealing with your colleagues as well as players, coaches and administrators that you are going to be interacting with as a journalist.

Do not forget that when you go out into the field and attend training sessions or press conferences for example, you will also interact with fellow journalists, many of whom you are likely to befriend, but some will become your rival; whether it be because they are from a competing media house, or for no good reason. The Flag Page information could be very beneficial to you in some of those instances.

Chapter Eleven
Alternative Sports Career Options

I promised earlier in this book to share with you how you can still be close to the action even without being an investigative reporter. That moment has arrived. Not everybody wants to be a reporter. Similarly, not everybody will become a reporter.

If you think that maybe reporting is not for you, or perhaps you are keen on an alternative career in sports journalism, this chapter is for you. In Chapter Two, we looked at Dictionary.com's definition of journalism, "the occupation of reporting, writing, editing, photographing, or broadcasting news or of conducting any news organisation as a business".[88]

Clearly, journalism is not just reporting although reporters tend to be the faces or the stars, much like presenters. In this section, you will meet four men who have made a career for themselves in sport outside of reporting. Get ready for a whirlwind adventure through camera operating, producing, photography and commentating in the words of some of the best in the business.

Television producer, Brian Gleeson has worked all over the world as a sports producer for some of the biggest television companies, like Sky Sports in the United Kingdom and BeIn Sports in Qatar. He is currently an executive producer for Virgin Media Television in his native Ireland.

South African Raymond Herbst describes himself as a television producer, but his work includes camera operating and video editing. He currently works as a freelancer and has previously covered several major tournaments for SuperSport.

---

[88] www.dictionary.com. (n.d.). Definition of journalism | Dictionary.com. [online] Available at: https://www.dictionary.com/browse/journalism?s=t.

Famous football commentator, Peter Drury will share insights with you from the commentary box. Englishman Drury has covered every FIFA World Cup since 1998 and every European Championships since 1996.

Finally, we have South African photographer, Lefty Shivambu. He started out covering school sport and has worked his way up through the ranks to now cover some of the biggest sports matches for major photography agencies.

What exactly does a producer do? It is a broad term in television terms as a producer at one channel might not necessarily perform the same tasks as a producer at another. For the purposes of this chapter, I shall highlight a producer who takes on the most responsibilities and Gleeson fits that description. In his own words, he explained what his job typically entails:

'The job of a sports producer will vary depending on whether you are producing news, live sport or a magazine style show. However, there are a few things that are required regardless of the content and those are planning, communication and decision making.

'It's up to the producer to decide what's happening, when, where and for how long and that takes a lot of planning. Ultimately the buck stops with you and you have to be prepared for all scenarios. Once your planning is done you have to be an excellent communicator, as now the studio crew, talent, transmission and numerous other departments need to get on board and understand your plan.

'Finally, especially in sport, you have to make decisions, hundreds of them, some tiny, some huge, but you must make them! When things start to get stressful or complicated everyone turns to the producer for the answers and the only wrong answer is not to have one. Sure, you'll make mistakes, but that's how you learn.

'I always use an analogy of an Orchestra to explain TV production. The producer has written the music, he or she is the Composer. They then give this music to the director who conducts all of the Crew/Orchestra in how best to play the music with the help of the Soloist/Presenters in order to entertain the audience.

'The one major difference is that at any point the producer may then rip up the music live on air and everyone will very quickly relearn the entire opera as they go along!'

Gleeson's advice for aspiring producers is to get yourself in the door, 'That's mission number one. Once you're in, make yourself indispensable. Learn as many roles as you can and what goes into them, so when you are a producer you know how all the moving parts work.

'Watch television with a critical eye as well as for enjoyment. If you loved something, think about why. If you hated something likewise. Be a sports fan and always remember your audience! Any time I produce something I try to imagine what I'd like to see if I were sitting at home. Do that and you won't go far wrong.'

It was not always Gleeson's ambition to become a television producer. He wanted to be a film director but has found producing to be just as much fun, 'Strangely being a television producer is not a million miles away. Especially as an assistant producer you will be asked to come up with a concept, film it, edit it and then put it on air, all with the goal of making your audience feel something.

'Sport, in particular, brings out incredible emotions and a well-made piece of television can make you laugh, cry or have the hair on the back of your neck stand up. There's no better feeling as a young AP than having an idea, seeing it through from concept to completion and then watching the reaction in person or online of complete strangers loving what you have created as much as you do.

'Very few will know or understand how much time, effort, collaboration and sheer bloody hard work has gone into perhaps just two minutes of television, but you will.'

Anyone who has ever taken the trouble to put together a three-minute clip for YouTube will know how much hard work audio and video production can be.

Raymond Herbst is also a television producer although when I first met him in 2009, he was working as a camera operator. Herbst's eyes were truly opened while covering cricket's Indian Premier League, FIFA Confederations Cup and FIFA World Cup in relatively quick succession.

He recalls, 'The IPL was the first gig I had. I didn't have to edit much. I just had to shoot thousands and thousands of little inserts. That was a baptism of fire and it was great. It wasn't even a career that I chose, it just sort of happened because that's where there was work to be done.'

Herbst covered the FIFA Confederations Cup soon thereafter and in between, continued to shoot news and magazine shows and then he found himself covering the FIFA World Cup in South Africa. He said that showed him what the sport industry was really like, 'You see auditoriums as big as lecture halls full of journalists and it's not like one part of the world, it was just this mesh of anywhere and everywhere in the world of people interested in football and I realised it was bigger than I could imagine.

'I'll never forget going to the first Argentina press conference in Pretoria. That was probably one of the defining moments of that tournament for me. I just looked at the first photo opportunity and it was just a mass of photographers and I didn't even realise there were so many people in this industry.

'I walked in and there was 100 press; just photographers, and then you look on the other side and there's another 100 cameramen. Obviously, Lionel Messi and Diego Maradona were huge for the South American news appeal and that's why there was anybody and everybody that had to be there, but it was just crazy. It was a great experience just to see the passion for sport.'

It is a real privilege to cover sport for a living. Never forget that. Herbst shared a funny story putting it into perspective, 'When I had to explain to my family members what I do as a job, they asked, "So you just do sports reporting? Who, where, what?"

'There is maybe one bulletin a day and they just couldn't grasp it but at that World Cup in 2010, there were entire channels and TV shows just dedicated to sport. It was so cool because you felt you had actually found a profession that is recognised worldwide.

'That was a defining moment for me and how I saw my career to realise that people actually take sports news seriously across the world. This is not just a willy-nilly job. From young people to guys that have been doing it 30, 40 years.'

His next big assignment was the 2011 Cricket World Cup in India, Bangladesh and Sri Lanka. I have already shared with you my own experiences of covering the 2012 Olympic Games as a non-rights holder. Herbst was fortunate enough to be part of a rights holder team.

However, he found the going tough too as he was expected to send daily reports to South Africa. He says, 'You don't have any support. It's a little bit of a different time zone and you're on your own with the journalists and you just have to produce as much as you can each day because the base team at home don't really know what you can or cannot do.

'You can pretty much say to them, "Sorry we couldn't do anything today" and they would have to accept it but it's a big opportunity for yourself and there's other people that should have or could have gone, so you just work yourself to death. Back then there wasn't good internet like now.

'You could hardly do a Skype. That was 2011, so 3G was just coming on the market and SuperSport had gone HD, so we were expected to deliver HD content to them, and it was harrowing to say the least. The logistics alone of getting around India was great fun, but it took forever.

'It didn't matter where you went. If you flew, drove, tuk-tuk, whatever, it just took such a large part of your day just to get to a function and it was sweltering hot. You film for four hours in the sun, then you can't really work there, so you go back to the hotel.

'You've done an eight-hour day's job but you haven't even done anything yet! Then you sit and edit and cater for magazine shows and news and all that. You have to quickly learn to manage yourself in this industry. I pride myself on never having missed a shoot or a deadline or a flight.

'You have to be passionate about the product or otherwise, you could literally just go on holiday. You could just excuse your way through it and say, "Sorry the logistics didn't allow us to do anything" and that's where the idea of being a professional dawned on me. This is not just a fun hobby. You either take this seriously or go do something else.'

Peter Drury is the world's foremost football commentator and an instantly recognisable voice to any football fan. Drury started in broadcasting in 1990. He has spent time at BBC, ITV, the Premier League and BT Sport. A dilemma that most aspiring commentators face is how to actually get into the business.

It can be a difficult process as Drury explains, 'Do everything you can to involve yourself in the business of sports broadcasting. That is to say, pester anyone who needs pestering that lives within a thousand-mile radius of you to allow you to get some experience.

'It's sometimes a soul-destroying spell in your life. In a pre-email age, I had piles and piles of letters of rejection for jobs I applied for and didn't get because frankly, I wasn't qualified to do them and of course, you couldn't be qualified to do them until you had the experience that wasn't forthcoming because you weren't qualified to get it and I know millions who are caught in that Catch 22.

'It's a case of persistence and in a way that persistence to an extent could act as a useful filter because in such a competitive industry you will only get there if you really, really want to get there. Half-heartedness will pull you up short and that's not even a criticism.

'It might be a useful jolt to show you actually what it takes to do this is not something that you really, really want to do in your life and that's fine. Move on and do something else.'

Contrary to some assumptions, a sports commentator does not simply arrive at the stadium on match day and start describing the action. Drury said there is significantly more to it than that, 'It does vary to quite a large degree depending on the type of match and where it falls in the season and so on.

'Broadly speaking it's a commentator's job, it was once said to me, to be in a position before a football match to know more about that football match than anyone else on Earth does.

'The aim of the game in terms of preparation is to make sure that every base is covered, that every possible eventuality is catered for, which if you look back too closely, can be a dispiriting thing because it could be that of the perhaps 6, 8 or 10 hours, or more, of preparation you do for each game, maybe 10% is going to be used.

'I go through every player and not just statistically but also importantly, where they are in terms of the news of the moment and what might happen to them next and how they're connected to this fixture and so on. All of that information a disciplined commentator should only use when it's relevant to the story.

'We've all been guilty in the past of having come up with a brilliant line, or so we believe, and using it for whatever reason because we've spent an hour working it out so you're damn well going to hear it whether you like it or not. Really, you should be disciplined about the use of the homework you've done so the vast majority of every game's homework goes to waste but it has to be there because what you've prepared might just happen.'

Drury shared that while on average, an eight-hour day prepares for a football match, there are often exceptions. Before sitting down to prepare for the 2019/20 Europa League final between Sevilla and Internazionale, he confessed he would have to research both teams from scratch.

'Given that I'm going to have to watch videos of them and work out which is which among the players and so on, that will be two whole days' worth, or maybe more, whereas if I'm doing Liverpool against Manchester United midseason, it still needs preparing player by player, but a lot of the base homework is in position already, so that might be four or five hours' worth.

'The challenge changes to one where you have to find something that you didn't say last week. And of course, statistics which I think are very much overused in television and radio these days, but nevertheless they seem to be part of the scenery and you have to be up to date with them.

'Roberto Firmino might well score three goals in the last four games and then he has four in the last five and then suddenly before you know it in a month's time, the statistic is Firmino hasn't scored for four games.'

Given the global exposure it enjoys, preparation for an English Premier League match between Liverpool and Manchester United can be relatively easy. I asked Drury what would happen if, for instance, he was assigned a hypothetical Africa Cup of Nations qualifier match between Burkina Faso and Benin.

Information regarding those players is considerably less easy to come by than those who are playing for Manchester United and Liverpool. Drury said it is a challenge that should be embraced, 'You start hammering the phones and finding someone who does know about them.

'I don't want to seem disrespectful to international football teams but I would compare it to perhaps doing a game in the very early rounds of the FA Cup where you're dealing maybe with a non-league team, an amateur team. Obviously, Burkina Faso is not an amateur team but the information available is similarly thin.

'Rather than going online to see how many goals and caps and whatever, it's a case of making personal relationships and speaking either to the people themselves if they become accessible, or at least to someone who knows them.

'I would try to get hold of the top commentator of Burkina Faso and say to him or her, "Please can we have an hour and talk through these players one by one", and because statistics are probably harder to come by, and rather dry and meaningless, I think in circumstances like that anyway, actually taking the trouble to come up with something a bit more personal and human interest would be your way to go about it.

'A bit of family background, a bit of something that has happened in their life will be preferable to what dry information there might be online i.e. that they are six feet tall, 24-years-old and played a dozen games for this club in Nigeria. So what? Everybody can look that up if they want to know it and they probably don't want to know it.

'In circumstances like that, I think you probably do have to go the extra mile and speak to people and truthfully, whatever the game, if you can speak to somebody and get that extra little titbit then that's your gold dust. It's lovely as a commentator to be able to tell the audience something that the audience doesn't already know and that is the challenge when it's Liverpool against Manchester United, because the audience already knows everything.

'There's nothing you can tell them to be perfectly honest and you sit there, and you think, "I'm a bit of a dummy here. What's the point of me? They all know who all the players are and if they want to know how many goals a player scored they can look it up", and it can be really exciting to do a game that doesn't fall into that category like Benin against Burkina Faso where you can find stuff out and actually genuinely educate your audience a little bit.'

With the preparation out of the way, it is time to head to the stadium for the actual match. It is not a case of arriving five minutes before kick off as Drury explains, 'I like to be there three hours before kick-off at least because I like the social experience actually and I think it's quite important.

'You bump into people, you speak to people and you find out little titbits and you hear the gossip and all that sort of thing, all of which can play into your day's work but also I do like to leave a lot of time for me – headspace room. For a four o'clock kick off on a Sunday, I get there at one o'clock, have lunch in the press room with colleagues, and chew the fat for a little while.

'The teams are published an hour and a quarter before the time with a 15-minute embargo for the likes of us, so we have some preparation time. In the period coming up to that 75 minutes from kick off, what tends to happen is that commentators will gather and pore over the team news together and have to work out the formations, or the likely formations, and then very quickly after that I like to scurry away, get up to the commentary position and prepare in two or three ways.

'One, I will literally write down what I will say about the team news. That's the key to assimilate it and work out what the story is, who should have been playing, who isn't, who should have been in, how they're going to line up because when the graphics come up, that is a 25-second set piece that you've got to deliver words over.

'So there's that and again, if you're watching a team that is unfamiliar, then that hour before kick-off is really important when the players are out there warming up in front of you, and I get the binoculars out and spend quite a long time looking at them one by one because if you get two or three players who look very similar that's your potential problem.

'For instance, one of the best-known clubs in the world, Manchester United, has its centre-halves Harry Maguire and Victor Lindelöf. Now you know what Maguire looks like. You know what Lindelöf looks like and so do I but from 50 yards away they are guys of similar height, darkish hair, similar skin colour, all of those things, and in a flash, you just might call the wrong name.

'You just might and there are countless examples of that. A lot of that period is looking for different colour boots. Who's got blue boots? Who's got orange boots? Who's got long sleeves? Who's got short sleeves? And all of those little demarcations that make the difference in terms of identification.

'There's scribbling to be done, there's maybe bits of recording for broadcasting that needs to be done and there's watching the players to be done and that more or less takes you up to four and you're on air.'

All broadcasters will eventually make mistakes. I once incorrectly called Real Madrid forward Gareth Bale "Christian Bale" during a live Champions League report on Al Jazeera. And you thought the only thing Batman does at night is fight crime!

Drury says any commentator who has worked for more than three years will eventually call out the wrong player's name. Once in Germany covering the 2006 World Cup, he found himself fatigued by a punishing schedule. He would be covering a match and then often on the same day travelling to cover a match the following day, and this pattern repeated itself for the best part of two weeks.

'One of the teams went 1-0 up and the same team scored again and I shouted: "Equaliser!" Because my head hadn't quite got to grips with who was in the lead and then to make matters worse having shouted: "Equaliser!" The goal was then ruled out,' he recalled.

Most commentators achieve a degree of fame for their witty one-liners. These moments are thoroughly prepared for, but yet unscripted, as Drury explained, 'There are certain things you can prepare. The words up to the start of a game you'd be silly not to be ready with those because you know what's gonna happen.

'Teams are going to walk out of the tunnel together. There is going be a roar from the crowd. They are gonna line up at the half-way line. They are gonna shake hands. Then you're gonna see the team graphics and then the game is gonna kick off.

'To me not to be prepared for what you absolutely know is going to happen is frankly ridiculous. That's like saying to Cristiano Ronaldo, don't bother practicing free kicks. You know you're going to get a free kick 20-yards out, so of course you spend hours preparing for that and you'd be unprofessional not to.

'Equally, when Liverpool were being presented with the Premier League trophy, I knew that at some point Jordan Henderson is gonna walk forward and pick up that trophy and show it to the world. You'd be stupid not to be ready for that. It's not a surprise. Anybody has the time to prepare for that.

'Between the first whistle and the last, you'd be equally stupid to try and script anything because live sport doesn't work according to a script. If you attempt to script it, it'll bite you. I'm not pretending it hasn't occurred to me that if someone scores, that'll mean this and that, so your preparation has to cover for that.

'If you know that Mo Salah's next goal is gonna be his 100th or Wayne Rooney's about to break Manchester United's scoring record, of course you've got to be ready for when he scores that goal. You cannot be ready for the precise context in which he will score that goal.

'If you try to write something down, you'll come up short and the best example I can give is the famous Sergio Aguero goal by which Manchester City won the league (in 2012).

'Now when I went to that game, I was prepared for the teams coming out the tunnel but I was also prepared, because Manchester City were almost certainly going to beat a very poor QPR team and win the league that day, for the final whistle to blow and Manchester City to be celebrating and then for Vincent Kompany to lift the trophy.

'Mercifully, I hadn't written a winning goal because I couldn't have known how that winning goal was going to come and to be honest, I'd assumed they would win 3-0 and there wouldn't be a winning goal.

'I sometimes go cold at the prospect of potentially having written that goal because whatever I'd written down wouldn't have done justice to that moment because it's one of those instinctive in-the-moment moments.'

Drury's advice to aspiring sports commentators is to only do it if you truly mean it, 'Don't do it because you think it will make you famous or in some sense well known because, I speak only personally here, only my opinion, to the extent that I am a little bit well-known, that's the bit I don't really like.

'I don't want that stuff, the fuss and whatever. I love going to live sport and articulating it. So, do it because you love the potential excitement of broadcasting live sport. That is the thrill. That is your day's work. Do it on the understanding that it's not just a free ticket. There is a lot of hard work involved.

'Do it on the understanding that it's going to require a thick skin at times because not everybody is going to like everything you do and sometimes that hurts but if you really mean it, and you're really up for it, it's completely worth all of that. It's a fantastically privileged position to be in and I wouldn't change it for the world.'

From television production, camera operating and match day commentary to traditional photography now. Lefty Shivambu started in 2000 and describes himself as "self-taught". Shivambu says the key to doing well as a sports news photographer is preparation.

By now, you should have picked up on that universal recommendation. 'Clean your cameras, get your cameras ready and look after your cameras and go early to the stadium,' said Shivambu.

One of the reasons it is important to arrive early according to Shivambu, is because even though you might have your press credentials, you might encounter a security guard who is not entirely familiar with the process. It might sound unusual but there is usually one security guard at every game who does not quite understand the media dynamics.

You might encounter that guy so arrive early to potentially engage in an unnecessary debate without losing too much time and still park your car. I have personally attended matches where the security guard would not allow me to park my car in the designated media parking zone. It happens.

Similar to Peter Drury, Shivambu likes to arrive at approximately 11:00 for a game kicking off at 15:00, 'By the time the game starts, I'm relaxed, and I can do exactly what I want to do. It's also very important to prepare and watch while the players are warming up. You capture those moments also.

'By the time the game starts, then you can shoot the action knowing that you already have stock pictures of the players and other individuals. Going to a game is not only about shooting the action. You must also do stock pictures. You don't just shoot two players tackling each other.

'You shoot the individual player, so that tomorrow when they talk about that player you have a picture of that player. It's not always about the game itself, but it's also about the other things so you make sure you have the picture of the actual player.

'You also set up your laptop, get a nice space for it, check your internet connection and these things are all very important as it takes a lot of the pressure away. If you're under pressure, you can't focus and if you can't focus, you're not going to deliver.'

Shivambu worked his way up from humble beginnings in South Africa's Limpopo province. 'I'm from Tzaneen. I was doing stuff for the local newspaper, *Letaba Herald*, but with a small "mik en druk"[89] camera. When I started in those days, you had to also do news and entertainment, as well as sport.

'I shifted myself to sport because it is more relaxed in terms of there not being much violence. Entertainment is also okay but sport you can learn something from. There can be a goal or there can be happiness and plenty of opportunities to get action shots so you can get really nice pictures.

'From Tzaneen, I moved to Pretoria and started doing school sports before starting to do stuff for the Premier Soccer League and (South Africa's national football team) Bafana Bafana. I pushed harder and Backpage Pix asked me to come and shoot stuff for them.

'I worked so hard that Kick Off magazine ended up saying to me they wanted me to come and help improve their soccer pictures so then I was hired by Gallo Images to do stuff for Kick Off,' he said.

In terms of being self-taught, Shivambu remembered reading a lot of books and asking for advice whenever he could. He started out covering school sport in Pretoria. He recalled, 'I thought if I go to the school sports like rugby, cricket and soccer I will build my career that way.

'In those days, rugby was the main thing for *Pretoria News* so I would go when Affies[90] was playing against Pretoria Boys High. It was always a big rivalry and it was good to go there. That's where you can build yourself. If you look at the kids now, most of them when they ask me questions about wanting to be involved in sports, and they want to shoot rugby or soccer or whatever, they mainly talk about the big stuff, like they want to go to Kaizer Chiefs or the Springboks, but I always say to them, it's always good when you're starting down there.

'That's when you're going to build your career nicely and you don't have any pressure. That's the most important thing because sports photography always has pressure in terms of what you are bringing to the table. If you go to the bigger teams, you will have a lot of pressure there.

---

[89] South Africanism. The best possible English translation is "point and shoot". It usually describes a cheaper less advanced camera designed for only the basics.

[90] Afrikaanse Hoër Seunskool. A famous boys-only high school in Pretoria.

'You are not going to learn a lot because there's no time to learn. All you have time for is to deliver and then you might see a seasoned photographer who gets nice pictures and that can actually demoralise you because you then think: "Why didn't I get that picture?" but you forget that you didn't want to start at the bottom and move your way up.

'Unfortunately, now it is difficult with the way life is because they also get challenged by social media. People want to see pictures of the best players on social media. They don't want to see the youngsters whereas when I was starting there was no social media. Even today, I am still motivated by school sports.

'I don't have a problem to go and shoot school sport. The advice I would give is about dedication and the love of sport and the love of what you're doing. That's the most important thing. Everybody can make it in life. Believe in God and believe in what you want to do.

'That's very important and also to believe in what you're doing. You must love your picture first. If you love your pictures, that's what's important. There are people that will say, "This picture you should have done so and so" but the most important person to love your pictures is you.

'You must believe in your work and be dedicated, and everything will come from there. But if you don't believe in your work, forget about other people believing in your work. It's good to ask for advice from senior people but you must remember that you must believe in your work.

'Do you really like that picture? Do you think that picture is good? I always believe in my work, but I look at other people's work and learn from them too. Believe in your work and be dedicated and you will do well. You can learn things from YouTube and you can improve yourself every day because when I was starting we still used film, so I couldn't see the picture, the shutter speed and so on.

'Sometimes, you just shot and hoped that the picture might work but then you had to go and work with that film in a dark room. But now, you can shoot and immediately see if the picture is good or bad. Don't worry about long lenses, standard lenses etc.

'When you go to a game, you will definitely come back with 10–15 pictures of good quality. Don't worry about someone sitting next to you with a 400mm lens when you only have a short lens. It doesn't matter what camera you have. With a short camera, you can also capture something.

'The big cameras and the big lenses will come but don't say: "Because I don't have these cameras I am not going to shoot the game". Go and shoot the game with that small camera and with that short lens. There's no way you cannot capture some of the best action. Also remember, the story is not only about the action.

'The story can be about Covid-19 now. If you are allowed to shoot a game, you can go and shoot an empty stadium or with the players inside that empty stadium without any fans. Don't forget to research beforehand. Maybe you are going to shoot Kaizer Chiefs v Mamelodi Sundowns.

'Do your research and visualise the game. Let's say it's the cup final. Look at the other games, look at how they celebrate, look at how the trophy is handed over and all that stuff. When I have to go to a game, especially a big game, I always visualise and imagine what kind of pictures I might come back with.

'I also look at the overseas way of doing things and then I think maybe when I'm at the game I might try to do similar stuff. I also look at the other photographers' work and go to the websites of other photography agencies and look at their presentation, so when I'm at the stadium I have an idea of what I might like to capture.'

There are many other jobs outside of reporting that a sports journalist can do but if they were to be highlighted, this book would never have been completed. Here you have read about producing, camera operating, commentating and photography and hopefully, it has given you some insight into the vast world of jobs available in sports journalism.

The advice that has been dispensed by our guests for this chapter is applicable to any career choice, really. Take it on board and you will be on the road to success. Further to that, you might want to incorporate one or more of these skills into your existing repertoire as the importance of being multi-skilled in the modern era grows more important by the day.

Chapter Twelve
Freelancing and the Advantages of Being Multi-Skilled

In this chapter, we are going to discuss freelancing, which is simply the act of providing services to a company as an independent contractor. Oftentimes, a freelancer provides services that are already provided by employed staff members but because the company has staff shortages or a need for more manpower for a particular period of time, they will choose to bring in a freelancer.

In other instances, freelancers can provide regular daily, weekly or monthly services and then typically send an invoice at the end of the billing period.

Freelancing offers its practitioners greater flexibility but be warned, it also offers the contractor the freedom to cut you off at short notice. Generally, freelancing is a great way to get started. In commercial radio, I started out as a freelancer.

Thankfully, my contracts were always renewed and then I secured full-time employment when I started my television career. However, when I joined Al Jazeera, it was initially as a freelancer. It was a risk I was prepared to take. My attitude was that I would work hard and try my best to impress the decision-makers and that way secure permanent employment.

Not everyone has that same philosophy though. There are many people that prefer to work on shorter-term contracts of 3–6 months, take a break, and then come back and do it all again. You will have to decide what is best for you. In this chapter, you will be introduced to British freelance journalist Paul Rhys, and become reacquainted with South African sports producer Raymond Herbst.

You will also again hear from Herbst's countryman Paul Kaye, the worldwide IRONMAN announcer, as well as Craig Norenbergs, former head of sport at Sky News Australia, the Australian Broadcasting Corporation Radio and Sky Sport in New Zealand.

Rhys is a well-established freelance journalist, Herbst has worked as a freelancer and entrepreneur and Kaye is a media generalist who has been on-air in radio and television as well as in management. All three men are multi-skilled and will share why they believe it is crucial to the modern journalist.

Rhys started out in newspapers but describes himself as a jack of all trades who always wanted to be in sport. I have already shared with you the importance of honing your skills at a community media house and/or through an internship. Rhys followed this path, working at a local newspaper at the age of 15 to gain experience.

He recalled, 'You can be sent out on anything and you've really got to get used to talking to people and teasing stories out of nothing. Some things will seem like utter drudgery, but you know you've got to write a story out of it. At university, I went from being a fairly talented but lazy student, to being a fairly talented but incredibly lazy student-journalist.

'I went along to the university newspaper in Manchester and wrote a couple of articles fairly half-heartedly. I wrote what I thought was a very good travel piece when I went to Sarajevo in 2000, for a student journalist, and got a big two-page spread on that, but I think I rested on my laurels a bit and concentrated on student life, drinking and being a fool.'

While he gained invaluable experience as a teenager, he found himself "drifting" as a young adult. He took a sales job in Sweden which brought him little joy, 'I was just sitting at a computer looking at figures and just thought, I can't do this. I've got to try and be a journalist.'

In a bizarre turn of events, his next move was to take up a job as a landscape gardener before he went to Paris to work as a barman – a job he had already done but that was when things changed for him.

'At my leaving drinks, my friend Catherine had cut out from the *London Evening Standard* an advert for a scholarship at the journalism school that was sponsored by *Trinity Mirror* which owns *The Daily Mirror* in England with lots and lots of regional newspapers and I kind of thought, *Yeah, it looks great but I'm going to Paris and it's going to be wild.* A week into Paris I realised I'd been an absolute idiot and I was too old to be an aimless barman in Paris,' said Rhys.

He found that very newspaper clipping in a sock drawer at his mother's house but found himself in a race against time. 'It was the day before the deadline, so I just ran to the computer in the spare room, updated my CV and just wrote this cover letter under deadline which turns out to be what we love!

'I sent it off, didn't hear anything for ages but eventually got called to an interview. Very much like me at the time, I worked out when the very last train I could get in the morning to go to the interview was and then decided I may as well go out for a few drinks, which turned out into quite a few drinks.

'I woke up after the last train had gone the next day, managed to get a shirt on and ran to the station and got there. I thought I was half an hour early, eventually I realised I wasn't. I ran trying to find the place and eventually got there all sweaty. Fortunately, they hadn't started and then we had to do a little test and a few writing exercises and then we kind of had to stand up and basically show off a bit in front of a panel of newspaper editors.

'I just remember a lot of the other candidates were editors of their former student newspapers and had actually done something with their budding journalist careers but were very nervous and I remember thinking they just weren't coming across well at all,' he recalled.

Despite being a bit hungover, a cocksure 23-year-old Rhys managed to impress the editors. They asked if he would take the position if offered it, but his response was anything but decisive. He said, 'I started playing hard-to-get and one of the editors on the South London Press said, "Well, you should" and I thought, *I may be in with a chance here.*

'I did get a place on this scholarship in Newcastle. It was a course that was under the two daily newspapers there in Newcastle, *The Journal* in the morning and *The Chronicle* in the evening. They paid us to do it and there was a job after the end of the course waiting for us. So, I can't think of what better course you could be on as a young journalist.'

The candidates were required to wear a suit and tie each day and were not allowed to be late. They also had short-hand lessons and Rhys eventually graduated and started work as a cub reporter on the *South London Press*, covering depressed areas of south London.

He remembers it being a great baptism of fire in journalism, 'I was immediately sent out on what was known as "death knocks". Someone would have a family member killed in a shooting, a knifing, or any other way, and you would have to go knock on the door of the family and try and persuade them to talk to the paper.'

While working as a young news reporter, Rhys met a local councillor who was fighting a racism case with the local council. This councillor was fobbed off on Rhys because he had a reputation as a loose cannon and the other reporters found him somewhat annoying.

It all paid off for Rhys, who had not yet given up on becoming a sports reporter. He recalled, 'He happened to be a sub-editor on the Financial Times or The Daily Telegraph and he got a job as the editor of the website for the Asian Games in Doha, Qatar in 2006.

'I think I was resigning myself to not becoming a sports journalist and I didn't really enjoy the news stories I was doing; stabbings and shootings and all sorts. He said, "Oh I didn't really think of it but I'll try and get you in", and I didn't hear anything for ages and then just suddenly one day got an email from the company doing the website in Qatar.

'Bear in mind, I was earning £12 000 a year in London, and he said "We're finishing our recruitment for Doha now. Would you like to come out here for three months at $5 000 a month or six months at $5 000 a month?" I took the job, loved Qatar as soon as I got there, and had a really great time.'

When you go out into the field as a reporter, you will not only interact with the players, coaches and administrators but you also spend a lot of time interacting with the journalists from other media houses covering these events. You will get to know them and even befriend some of them, even if you are trying to out-scoop one another.

It was in this setting that Rhys' next opportunity presented itself. 'I was sent out to cover one of the opening events and happened to be sitting next to Joanna Gasiorowska of Al Jazeera English's sports department. I got chatting to her and she put me in touch with the head of their website and I got interviewed for a job at Al Jazeera and accepted for it,' he says.

While waiting for his residency permit application to be successful, Rhys spent time covering the Olympic Games in Beijing and doing work as a national news agency reporter in England, travelling the country, knocking on doors and even spent time outside Bob Geldoff's mansion trying to get an interview. He then became the head of the sports section of Al Jazeera's website.

Rhys says, 'There was only one other person and me working on it at the time so it's not as amazing as it sounds. I was sitting with the sports team and kind of saw what they were doing and wanted to be part of it after seeing how exciting the whole TV journalism process was. I was lucky enough that they sent a huge team to South Africa for the football world cup in 2010 and they sent me to cover it for the website which is amazing really.'

Rhys says it was while in South Africa that he began experimenting with his equipment when his adventurous side got the better of him, 'I was sitting in the office in Johannesburg writing blogs and I just thought I can't sit here for six weeks in an office in Joburg.

'I've got to get out and see the country and try and report on the country, so I just hired a car and took a little flip camera with me and just drove around the country trying to film little packages, just trying to emulate what I'd seen from the TV output from Joanna and Andy Richardson for example.

'I had an amazing experience on the road going to townships, going to football matches, covering different aspects of things and almost getting beaten up by English hooligans. That was the most danger I had encountered travelling South Africa on my own, was coming up against English hooligans.

'I edited a lot of little packages out of it and then from that stage, I just tried to slowly invest in better equipment and did the same kind of thing at the Rugby World Cup in New Zealand and got my first packages on air doing that.'

While it might sound like a dream-come-true scenario, Rhys admits it was far from perfect in those early days, 'I look back on it now and it is dreadful stuff but you know, you have to do that dreadful stuff before you get to slightly less dreadful stuff and slightly less dreadful than that.'

Rhys then came close to becoming an on-air sports news presenter when Al Jazeera held pilot sessions looking for a new presenter. Although he missed out, he applied for a position as a news output producer and got it but, he says, he soon realised after a few sessions training as an output producer, that he missed the sports department too much.

'I went with my tail between my legs and thought I might just actually lose my job altogether and said, "I don't want to be an output producer, I want to be in sport". I'd already been offered the job and signed the contract.

'They could have just told me to sling my hook that day, but they actually said, "Okay we'll make you an output producer on sport". Sarah Worthington was head of output at the time and I thought that was amazingly kind, so I got to train under people like Andy Richardson and James Pratt who was the head of sport at the time and got to know how to put out a sports bulletin.'

While all this was going on, the urge to use his camera would not go away as he explains, 'I tried to go out and shoot more packages and my thought was that I was never going to get sent out with a cameraman when they can send out Andy Richardson or Joanna Gasiorowska.

'It just wasn't going to happen, so I just thought since that's usually a three-person send, lots of flights and lots of per diems, why don't I make myself a cheap option? Just me and my camera VJ-ing. So that was my aim and I went to the Africa Cup of Nations in 2013 in South Africa.

'One or two of my packages were dreadful and I actually got pulled off air which gutted me at the time. I felt so resentful at the person who pulled it off the air, but they were totally right.'

The seed had been sown though and Paul Rhys the Freelancer was just one step away from becoming reality. He says, 'I thought to really go somewhere with this, I've got to leave my really nice job at Al Jazeera and actually go out in the field somewhere because however much I slowly improved, I wasn't going to improve quickly so I decided to move to Paris and invested in better kit and from there just sort of slowly improved, shooting more and more stuff.'

While he was no longer based at the headquarters in Doha, he now found himself in continental Europe and available to cover stories in that region at a minute's notice. That is what puts a freelancer at an advantage, he says, 'It's a lot easier to get sent to stories when you're already out there, than what it is to get sent from Doha.

'I made a lot of mistakes along the way, huge mistakes. I still make mistakes now but not quite so big and I just enjoy the whole process. I enjoy shooting, scripting, editing. I even enjoy my piece-to-cameras now and I get a big buzz out of it.'

You would have noted how Rhys has skilled himself as a cameraman, editor and scriptwriter as well as an on-air presenter and correspondent. Remember that the competition for journalism jobs is steep, so the ability to be flexible and versatile is something that can only be advantageous.

In May 2020, Microsoft announced it would not renew the contracts for dozens of news production contractors working at MSN and planned to replace them with artificial intelligence. Roughly 50 employees found themselves out of work.

One of the fired workers complained, 'It's demoralising to think machines can replace us but there you go.'[91] Consider what Rhys does and ask yourself if he could easily be replaced by a robot?

While I personally think it is unrealistic to expect one person to do the work of four or five, the harsh modern reality is that one-trick ponies are increasingly out of favour. The more you can offer a company the better but as a freelancer, it is almost like having super powers.

I want to bring in a quote from Yusuf Omar, co-found of Seen, 'I think the greatest skill that a journalist can have is the ability to acquire more skills. I think the days of singularly being a videographer, or photographer, producer, editor, is gone. You've got to have a holistic skill set or you have to be bloody brilliant at the one skill that you do.'

No matter how much you dislike the idea of having to become good at something you do not have much enthusiasm for, it is best you embrace it. Rhys shares the story of a friend of his who saw the winds of change blowing a decade ago, 'He was on my course in Newcastle as a newspaper journalist.

He started working for a newspaper in Cardiff, Wales – the *South Wales Echo* I think, and probably about 10–12 years ago, they started sending him out with a camera to do little video segments while writing for the paper and a lot of the old school guys refused to do this, saying, "It's a separate job. We've got to resist this".

'Maybe in one respect, they were right because people have lost their jobs because less money is being spent on photographers in local and national papers. But he saw already back then the slashes in budgets at newspapers and he knew he could take a stand, or he could go with the flow and just lean in to it as they say, and he did.'

In terms of his own skill set, Rhys says it was not something he was ever asked to develop but it came from his own initiative, 'I just thought I had to make myself flexible and cheap. I thought it was the only way I was going to go a bit higher in the pecking order.'

Rhys says if the budgets were a little lower in a particular month or there was a need for someone to cover a different aspect of a tournament, and he was

[91] The Seattle Times. (2020). Microsoft is cutting dozens of MSN news production workers and replacing them with artificial intelligence. [online]Available at: https://www.seattletimes.com/business/local-business/microsoft-is-cutting-dozens-of-msn-news-production-workers-and-replacing-them-with-artificial-intelligence/.

already there, then he became an attractive option given the way he had set himself up.

The danger of being a jack of all trades but master of none is something Rhys says he has experienced personally, 'I think I could be a much better cameraman than I am now. I think I've made the main improvements in the last year or so. In fact, just before I'd gone on a five-day shoot which I'd been trying to pitch for about three years.

'I was playing a rugby league match in the Czech Republic and I split my head open with a deep scar three days before I was going to have to shoot a piece-to-camera on an expensive send for Al Jazeera in the north of Sweden, which was absolutely gutting but I just thought if I'm going to look patched up with horrendous makeup over a bloody wound on my piece-to-camera, I have to at least make sure the rest of it is as nice as possible.

'It was actually only then that I started studying camera work and how to get the best shots. I think I was making step-by-step improvements anyway, just maybe in shooting style and editing, but I didn't really get to know my camera until about a year ago.

'It is great being multi-skilled but you still need to try and go a bit deeper into the skills. I think multi-tasking is definitely an asset but each one takes away from the other and we're not designed particularly to be multi-taskers either so it's a lot of work to keep the quality high.'

While it can be very rewarding when it all comes together, Rhys warns that the process of being a multi-skilled one-man show has its own stresses and that wherever possible, he prefers working in a team, even if it is just one additional member.

'If things are going badly, you don't have anyone there to lighten the mood. You can't joke about it. All you can do is curse yourself and get in a sweaty mess so it's more fun when you're working with someone.' The other advantage an additional team member gives you on a shoot is having someone there to talk to your interviewee and keep them comfortable while you are setting up your camera and audio equipment.

Raymond Herbst and I first met during the 2009 Indian Premier League cricket tournament. Herbst is skilled at camera operating, video editing and producing. He believes being multi-skilled is not even negotiable anymore. 'I'm not saying you have to be a cameraman, for a lot of people it's just not their jam but you have to know what goes into it.

'I've worked hard with European crews on the golf and they've actually changed the whole way that they do television production. You don't become a professional at something right away. You become a very skilled operator so it's junior producing, producing, field producing and then they move you into a technical department where you have to edit, and they even make you do basic camera work just so when I'm talking to you and I say, "I need you to do this and that", I won't have to explain to you that the sun is behind your head and I can't see your face.

'TV is just too integrated. I might have to ask you to shoot a press conference while I try and go poach a shot outside. You don't have to be an expert. You just have to hold the frame. I've had to produce, shoot, interview, lay voice and guide tracks just as a basic because it's just critical.

'You can't see it as "I'm not a cameraman. I'm not a sound guy". You have to see it as an awesome opportunity. It's free knowledge. It's a crash course and TV is great because of the relentless pace. I still think it's a great platform for people to learn.'

Herbst added that the skills you learn in television production will give you an edge if you decide to try your hand at things like YouTube, 'A lot of people are learning how much goes into three minutes. Try and do a three-minute vlog. They put it on and speak into a mic for three minutes and it's hellishly boring and they see people are only watching the first ten seconds and they ask why.

'It's because they only got to the good stuff after three minutes, where we know how to do that because we had old producers drum on about hooks and whatever. If you don't have the mind-set that you're going into TV to learn, then don't even bother.

'Editing, audio technology, recording equipment and the way people are doing stories changes every day. I look at stuff I produced in 2010 and I look at what I'm doing now and the old stuff doesn't feel right and it's because I've learnt so much and the equipment allows you to do things and you're just learning all the time so you'd be a fool to come into the industry and think you're going to be a news anchor and that's it. You're just wasting your time. Even Oprah didn't work like that. She did everything.'

It was while attending the NBA All-Star game in New Orleans that Herbst spotted a sign that really resonated, 'They have an NBA media room which is like their internal media, and so first and foremost before anybody else gets an interview, the NBA gets their stuff. There's this massive road sign with a cross through the middle that says, "That's not my job" and that is critical for TV.

'That was one of the best signs I've ever seen. Why wouldn't you give that person a cable? I know a lot of old guys will say you're not the lighting guy so you don't touch the cable but in today's day and age everybody's got to be able to help because you never know when you might be ill, or you can't be there for the day or whatever. It shouldn't be a bad thing. It should be a great thing that you can do anything in this industry.'

Herbst's advice to anyone considering freelancing, or already in that sphere, is to never compromise on your equipment, 'you have to always invest in your tools which is your cameras, your laptop etc. If I'm working with you as a freelancer, you hire me and my edit takes slow because my equipment is junk, I just look tardy and my things look old.

'It might be bad that people see it that way, but it makes a massive impression if your equipment works well and you deliver a product very quickly. I've invested almost too much money into my equipment just so it's not a time-sucker. One hour's delay one day is fine. One hour every day for seven days and now you've lost a workday.

'People quickly start second-guessing you if your equipment is second rate. They'll be asking why they're paying you and what you use your money on. Is it your lifestyle? It costs money but invest in your equipment. It's the best thing I've ever done. It really sets you apart.'

Paul Kaye started as a radio presenter at Stellenbosch University's then-Radio Matie in 1988. A year later, he was their head of broadcasting, before joining Radio Goeie Hoop which became Good Hope FM. He started hosting weekend shows but then also sport and by putting his hand up for every opportunity, he was soon the go-to stand-in host.

He later became the programme manager and then the station manager. Five years later, he became the global marketing manager for a software firm but he did not enjoy that, so he left to join *Runners' World* and *Bicycling* magazines. He was eventually promoted to publisher and then he moved into digital publishing.

Kaye is currently a worldwide IRONMAN announcer travelling the world covering IRONMAN events. He is the very epitome of a jack of all trades. On being multi-skilled, Kaye advises to put your hand up for everything, 'I put my hand up for any stand-in that came along.

'I put my hand up to do the sport. I even read news when it was required. I did weather when it was required. When we were doing outside broadcasts, I helped the OB technician and in those days in the early 1990s we didn't have active speakers, we had passive speakers with magnets the size of the sun so carrying a speaker felt like you were carrying a ton.

'Whether it was a beach challenge or a fun run, whatever it was, by putting my hand up for everything and being willing to do everything and leaving my ego at the door, I learnt a lot but in the process of learning a lot I also showed I had other talents.

'If you look at the sort of YouTube and podcasting you're seeing, there are a lot of people there who are relying on the digital technology to do everything for them. They're not making sure they're using the right mic and using it properly, so you see poor mic technique, or too much head room on the video camera, not getting the light right.

'A little bit of technical know-how really, really helps you too because it helps you make the best of what you're good at so if you've got a good voice, don't stand miles away from the microphone. Get a little bit closer and use more of your voice.

'Put your hand up for everything, be a sponge, work your butt off, learn as much of the trade as possible because that learning helps you specialise ultimately. It will give you many more arrows in your quiver to help you to hit the target you want to hit.'

Former head of sport at the Australian Broadcasting Corporation Radio, Sky News Australia, and Sky Sport in New Zealand, Craig Norenbergs also has some crucial advice that applies to being multi-skilled. It should be seen as non-negotiable according to him.

'If you've seen what has recently happened to the industry everywhere, at least in the western world, it's the multi-skilled people in the newsrooms who will survive. These days with the accountants looking over the books and more and more businesspeople buying into the business of media, they are looking to shave costs wherever they can.

'If you're a good all-rounder, you're going to keep your job. You want to build a career. Presenting jobs are a flash in the pan if you're just a presenter, a one-trick pony, but production jobs or being a good all-rounder will pay for a career and a career gives you a house, education for your kids and your retirement.

'The worst kind of presenters are the ones who've never produced. They've never been in the trenches. There's longevity in being able to produce, and write, and work in the field and be a journalist. If you're just a presenter, or if you're just a producer, that's not good enough anymore, but if you can voice stuff, if you can go out in the field, if you can put together a rundown, if you can do teambuilding and look after teams, that gives you longevity.

'My advice for anyone starting out in the business is to be the best all-rounder that you can. If you're at university, I'd certainly look at trying to be the best all-rounder. Don't just sit there thinking, "I'm going to be the best presenter one day", or "I'm going to be a correspondent one day".

'I remember doing a course on the editing system Media Central and one of the correspondents just didn't want to do it because she said, "I'm a correspondent. I don't need to know this", but I remember thinking, "I need to know. This makes me a better all-rounder". If you can voice, write and edit, you've got it made in this business, which isn't to say that some technology might not come along in five years and change it all again.'

Norenbergs said when he took the Sky News Australia job, the channel was just starting up and he had to hire a team from scratch. Many who he approached rejected him. It was a golden opportunity missed he says, 'It was funny the number of people I had initially approached who said "no" because they said they wanted to work for Fox Sports.

'It was probably the worst decision they ever made because they actually had a head of sport coming to them. They were working in radio and I understood it was their dream to work at Fox, but they could have taken the job with me, gained television experience and then applied. As it was, the people that I started hiring are now big stars in Australian television because they earned their chops with me.'

Whether freelancing or full-time employed, if the head of sport approaches you, recognise the uniqueness of the opportunity and think very carefully about rejecting the offer.

Paul Rhys echoes that advice, arguing the most important thing for a freelancer starting out is to be available, 'Don't say no. Once you're extremely established, "No" comes a little bit easier to the people who are asking you to do things.

'When you've not got a lot of experience and you get an opportunity just grab it and I think what I've done for most of my career is gone for it and been there and just done it and often at my own expense because I just thought it was too good an opportunity to miss.

'On one occasion, and this can be a lesson because it was extremely painful for me at the time, I said no to something that came up quite early on while being a freelancer and I realised very quickly afterwards that it was an extremely stupid decision and it took me a long time to get over it.

'If at all Earthly possible, if you're asked, just do it. If you're thinking of saying no, have a really long think about how you really might feel about letting that opportunity go and having people remember that you said no.'

You will often hear stories about how people have done certain freelance jobs, be it correspondence, deployments, and even jobs that are more entertainment-related like voice-over work and master of ceremonies duties. What you seldom hear is how they got those jobs and even more rare, is finding someone who will tell you how to get those jobs.

I asked Rhys to share with us how he goes about securing work as a freelancer and thankfully for you, he was happy to be candid. 'I think because I came straight from Al Jazeera with the intention of working as much as possible for Al Jazeera, and I was friends with some of the people I was pitching to and on the news side at least I was known to the people I was pitching to, and I had an Al Jazeera email address made it a lot easier.

'Of course, I had to do the work to be in that position to have those contacts and have people have some faith in me but knowing people is a huge step forward. I think if you can get yourself in that position where you already know people and you can get some work, that can maybe stop a lot of rejections but other than that it's a lot of cold stuff,' he says.

Rhys rates Al Jazeera as the best news channel in the world to work for, 'I'm not saying it's perfect, but you have so much editorial freedom. It's really rare that what I've edited is changed when it goes out. In news, we have more script editors, but they tend to improve it and it is great freedom and I love the reporting that the channel does and it's great to be in that.'

While Rhys has done a lot of his freelance work for Al Jazeera, he has also contributed to the Associated Press and Reuters. In terms of real actionable advice Rhys suggests, 'I think you've got to take in the same attitude as when you're ringing up a contact or trying to get a story.

'You've got to ring up, be friendly, say who you are, and I think if you're trying to get work don't take up too much of their time, be to the point, and then if you don't hear back, remind them politely later on but don't be a Crazy. Don't be someone that they just dread seeing an email from in their inbox or hearing a phone call from. You've got to tread that line between being pushy and putting yourself out there and not being a pain.'

The age-old question is how often should you email or phone someone when looking for a job? There is no perfect answer and it probably depends on the other person's personality type. The chances are extremely high that you do not know the personality type of the person you are emailing or phoning.

If there is a genuine deadline attached to what you are pitching, then it makes sense for you to contact them more often but beyond that all you can try to do is avoid being annoying. I was once contacted on LinkedIn by a guy who wanted to write for my sports news website, *The Sports Eagle*.

I gave him my email address and he promptly mailed me his CV and an example of his previous work. Within five minutes of sending the email, he sent me another message on LinkedIn to see if I had received the email. I courteously replied in the affirmative before he replied, "Have you read through it?"

While there is no perfect answer to the acceptable frequency of email follow-ups, whatever you do, do not be like that guy. I found it annoying and I tend to have a higher level of tolerance for such things. You have to accept that there are going to be people that are not going to reply to your email or phone you back. The best you can do is move on or try again at a later stage. That is later as in a week or month, or six months, or a year, not five minutes.

Rhys has some additional advice for freelancers. He says it is about maximising your opportunities, 'One of my first sports journalism gigs was the Rugby World Cup in 2007 in France working on a news service at the event. I've kept that up and that can also help to be sent somewhere by someone and then if your contract ends before the tournament, stay there, because then you're suddenly available for other people.

'A few times, I've gone to a Rugby World Cup, or gone to something for the first half of the tournament on a contract, and then stayed to be a cameraman or a reporter if someone else wants me. That's a good way to piggyback two things. That's not the same as trying to get a day's pay out of someone and then selling your stuff to someone else.

'You've got to be very careful with that kind of thing, but if you can get sent somewhere by one person, finish your duties with them, and then stay there, that's a good way to do it.'

I have done something similar. When I was sent to London to cover the 2012 Olympic Games for eNCA, I also provided Bloemfontein-based radio station OFM with daily 60-second reports. I arranged to record those very early in the morning, so that way the radio station had them in time for their breakfast show but also by doing it that way, it did not interfere with the work I had to do in London for eNCA.

Crucially, there was no conflict of interest there, which is what Rhys was warning against. Do not go to an event as a freelancer for TV Station A and then in between provide TV Station B with content. Believe me, it will not be long before you struggle to sell your work to any TV station!

I asked Rhys why he chose the freelancing path. He said it was mostly because he wanted to be out in the field more. 'It was one of the packages I'd shot in South Africa at the World Twenty20 cricket in 2007.

'After I'd shot and edited it and seen it go out on air, even though I'd had some terrible mistakes from the production end, I went and sat in the sun at Newlands, watching South Africa v Pakistan I think, and I just had such a euphoria after shooting this package.

'I just thought, this is it, this is what I want to do. As it turns out that was the package that got pulled! But the feeling I got out of it was that this was what I needed to do and as soon as I stopped enjoying living in Doha, I thought that was the time for me to do it. I had to get in the field, I had to move to Europe. I got myself some kit and thought, "Let's see what I can do". At that point, I really wanted it.'

Full-time employment provides a security that freelancing does not but this is not something that bothers Rhys too much, 'If I can briefly give myself some praise, I think I have been brave in pursuing what I want from my career and I think that really helps.

'Don't get me wrong, I've had visions of myself in a gutter having messed up my freelance career, but I think the wanting it and wanting to pursue certain things has won out in the end. The projected enjoyment and fulfilment has to win over the feared pain.'

Finally, be protective of your ideas as a freelancer. Not everyone you meet in this industry wishes you well. When I moved from radio to television, I took a significant pay cut and to supplement my income, I took a few freelance magazine writing jobs. I was happy to share this information with one of my colleagues.

As it turned out a few months later, he was writing for one of those magazines and I was out of favour. I thought about mentioning his name in this book, but I made peace with his betrayal a long time ago. Let it be on his conscience I say. Further to that consider the following tweet:

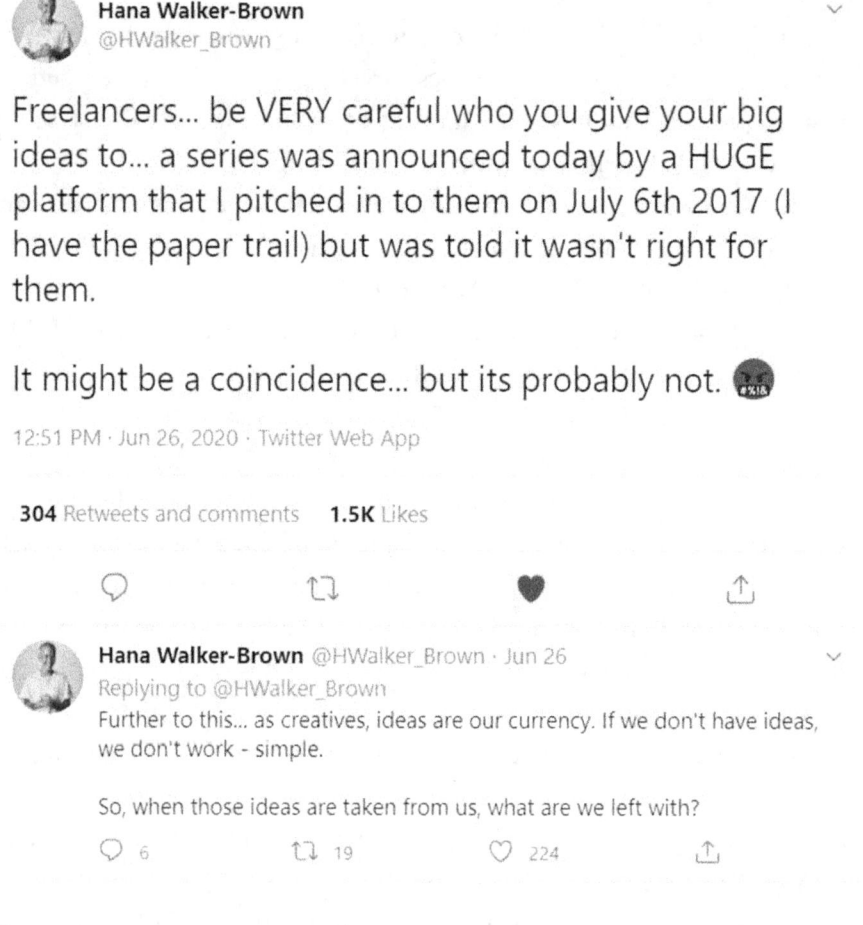

Hana Walker-Brown
@HWalker_Brown

Freelancers... be VERY careful who you give your big ideas to... a series was announced today by a HUGE platform that I pitched in to them on July 6th 2017 (I have the paper trail) but was told it wasn't right for them.

It might be a coincidence... but its probably not. 😡

12:51 PM · Jun 26, 2020 · Twitter Web App

304 Retweets and comments   **1.5K** Likes

Hana Walker-Brown @HWalker_Brown · Jun 26
Replying to @HWalker_Brown
Further to this... as creatives, ideas are our currency. If we don't have ideas, we don't work - simple.

So, when those ideas are taken from us, what are we left with?

6   19   224

Hana Walker-Brown and I were not the first, and certainly will not be the last, who have been blindsided by unscrupulous operators fronting as friends. Guard your ideas with everything you have got.[92]

---

[92] Twitter. (n.d.). https://twitter.com/hwalker_brown/status/1276453109313740807. [online] Available at: https://twitter.com/HWalker_Brown/status/1276453109313740807 [Accessed 4 June 2020].

Freelancing is not for everyone. Many people prefer the security of having a steady income through full-time employment, but it is important to give you an insight into what life can be like for a freelance sports journalist. There are thrills to be had for sure. In the next chapter, we shall delve into a role that requires even more bravery – sports media entrepreneurship.

Chapter Thirteen
Starting Your Own Sports Media Business

As you now know, freelancers are entrepreneurs in the sense that they are selling a service but for a real thrill, you might want to consider starting your own media business. In this chapter, I shall introduce you to multiple award-winning South African sports journalist, Junia Stainbank who quit his sports reporter job at eNCA to found African Sports Content Network (ASCN).

If you have worked in the television sports news space, you will be familiar with the agency SNTV (Sports News Television). Agencies cover a large variety of sports and news content that is accessible via a subscription service. All major news channels subscribe to services like these.

An organisation might be limited geographically, or resource-wise, but thanks to these agencies, they are able to broadcast content they have not been able to directly cover.

Nobody starts a business without having some sort of background knowledge. Most people work in an industry first before making the jump. Stainbank was studying in New York City at the Lee Strasberg Theatre and Film Institute before he found himself in the world of sports media for the first time.

The self-confessed introvert recalls, 'I struggle with starting conversations, it makes me very anxious, but I found that one of the easiest ways to relate to people was through sport. New York being the melting pot of cultures and nationalities that it is, I'd bump into an Australian and we could start talking about cricket, and I could do that.

'It was an easy ice-breaker. I'd bump into an American and we could speak about the Knicks, the Giants, and the Yankees and so on. If I bumped into an Englishman, we could speak about rugby.'

He soon found himself frequenting sports bars in the Big Apple and a job in sports writing followed. Stainbank says, 'I had a friend who ran a digital blog in

New York and he asked me to write something on Cesc Fabregas and that was the first article I ever wrote.

'It was the season where he was the only good thing at Arsenal. When I got back to South Africa, I realised that I had fallen a bit out of love with the dramatic arts and I needed to engage with something.'

Weekends spent with his friends watching sport triggered an idea to turn their frank conversations into a web series called *Fool Time*. He says that was the start of his sports journalism career. Stainbank produced the show and wrote articles for *Fool Time's* various social media pages.

After 18 episodes, the group of friends ran out of money and finding sponsorship was challenging given the colourful language often used during the conversations. Even so, he used his work at *Fool Time* as the basis for his CV.

'I started sending it out and Guy Hawthorne (head of sport) was the one guy who responded and he gave me a shot at the desk at eNCA based on what we had recorded, what we had shot, me producing it and also what I had written for the blog. I spent six months at the desk and then Guy moved me up to reporting,' he says.

That was quite a meteoric rise, but you have already heard from others in this book that being multi-skilled and putting your hand up for things is an asset. Stainbank went from recording a show with his friends for YouTube, to being a desk producer, to being a reporter in a relatively short space of time. That speaks to ambition but also hard work and being available.

Stainbank would go on to win the SAB Sports News Reporter of the Year award three years in a row for his excellent work at eNCA. That is the same award I won in 2009 although that was the lone occasion I was to win that accolade. Thanks for making me look bad in my own book, Junia!

He did not actually leave eNCA with the intention of starting ASCN straight away. There was a deeper meaning to his resignation. 'I had it in the back of my mind during that period, giving it some thought, writing down some notes, very slowly expanding the idea in my mind but in reality, I actually just left because I was depressed. I'd left for my own mental health. Every day felt like I was going to have an anxiety attack. It was not sustainable,' Stainbank says.

One issue that got him down was the lack of opportunity to report on the stories that he most wanted to cover. That is one of the downsides of being a general reporter. At most, 24-hour broadcast news houses a sport reporter will not have a beat but instead function as a general reporter.

While it is the accepted model, there are very few sports journalists that possess the kind of expert knowledge required for that kind of role. You will have to just get on with it as best you can, but a niche is where you can best distinguish yourself.

Remember how I shared with you earlier in the book how I carved a niche for myself with boxing and tennis? Stainbank did this with women's sport. If you can put yourself in this position, you might get to cover the stories closer to your heart more often, but you will still be forced to cancel interviews with your contacts from time to time because your editor assigns you to a supposedly bigger story. Be mindful of that.

Stainbank says, 'I covered a few Banyana Banyana (South Africa's national women's football team) and women's Proteas (national cricket team) stories and there was a women's Proteas story I did where Momentum (insurance company and team sponsor) and Cricket South Africa awarded seven or eight professional contracts for the first time.

'I went to a training session at SuperSport Park where I went to get some soundbites. I spoke to Mignon Du Preez (then-captain) and the training session ended. I had my training viz. I had my bites and we were walking back to the car with the camera operator and Chloe Tryon (all-rounder), who was walking to the dining hall asked if we were hungry.

'I really wasn't, but I wanted more access and she said, "Come in". So, we sat at the table having lunch and across the table was Mignon. Chloe was on my right, Dané Van Niekerk (recently retired captain) was at the table, I think Suné Luus (current captain) had recently debuted and she was around, and you are never going to get that in the men's game. We chatted and we spoke off the record and then we got up and we left.'

That kind of access was something he realised he was unlikely to get from the men's game, and not just cricket but other sports too. He compares getting a quote from top flight football or rugby players to extracting teeth but it also brought about an epiphany.

'I started realising that I might be the only reporter there covering their training sessions, so that opened up all these doors and opportunities for me to really get in with these athletes and speak to them on a level that AB De Villiers won't speak to me on, because with all due respect to AB, he's had years and years of being taught that the media is the enemy for some reason.

'I started covering women's sport consistently and carved out a niche for myself in that regard and I started feeling somewhat responsible for them and I loved that feeling. I loved the accountability that comes with that. I loved the feeling that my coverage might contribute to a sponsorship that could change the trajectory for an athlete as opposed to just being for coverage's sake.'

The desire to cover these athletes became unquenchable, 'As I got more invested in women's sport, my expectations of what we should be doing grew. I was quite comfortable in the beginning just covering this or that and getting some stories on Prime (eNCA's terrestrial channel eTV's flagship evening news bulletin) that reflected the excellence of this athlete or that athlete, but the more you do it you realise we could do even more.

'We've actually got enough resources to do more. There's enough smart people in this newsroom to do more and I'd push and I'd push and I'd try to expand the diary to include more women's sport wherever I could but it hit a wall at some point.'

That wall was not only a barrier to covering more women's sport. He hit an editorial brick wall shortly before the 2016 Olympic Games. Stainbank found it curious that South Africa's telecommunications parastatal, Telkom, used Usain Bolt as the face of their campaign to promote the Games, especially since they were also a sponsor of South Africa's Olympic team.

At the time, Wayde Van Niekerk was the 400 metre world champion and a favourite to take the gold medal in Rio de Janeiro. Why, Stainbank wondered, would a South African state-owned company prefer Bolt over one of their own?

He says, 'It just didn't make any sense, so I did a story on sponsorship that got me called into the passage of the Joburg office called "Management Mile" and I got grilled about my intentions. The fact is that the comms person at that major telecoms parastatal was someone who was well known to those people on "Management Mile" and this was the person that I needed to get a response from on camera and they weren't crazy about it and I remember being told it was a "whiny story".'

Stainbank was told that his story left an after taste of people whining for attention they had not earned. After explaining his position, he was told that if someone like Van Niekerk wanted to be the face of the campaign, he should pull up his socks and perform.

That might well be the height of irony considering Van Niekerk was the reigning world champion and the first sprinter in history to run the 100 metres in under 10 seconds, 200 metres in under 20 seconds and 400 metres in under 44 seconds. Moreover, he was widely considered the favourite for the Olympic gold medal and even seen as a possible successor to Bolt as the poster boy of world athletics.

Stainbank felt vindicated two months later when Van Niekerk became the Olympic champion by running the fastest 400 metres time ever (43.03 seconds) and became a mainstream media sensation in South Africa but it also further motivated him to go it alone. 'The confines of mainstream media would always prevent me from doing as much as I thought we could and that started to really weigh on me,' he says.

Starting a business is a daunting prospect. It requires quitting your secure day job and stepping into the great unknown. It is not just setting up the parts of the business you know well but also the intimidating administrative process. Stainbank says, 'There was a study that was done on the best countries in Africa to start a new business.

'I think Morocco came out on top and that just comes down to how a government facilitates the ease of doing business for new and small businesses. South Africa did not rank very highly on that list and once you're in it for a while you realise why. I spent a long time trying to get this business off the ground.

'My friend Christopher is the first person I bounced this idea off and when we were speaking at the beginning of 2018, he said, "So how much time do you think you're going to need?" and I said two-and-a-half years and Christopher now says to me it's bonkers how accurate I was.

'At the time, he said two-and-a-half years is a long time and I was going to go so broke and there would be no way I could keep my apartment and I said, "Yeah, you're absolutely right but I think two-and-a-half years is really what's needed".

'Taking as long as we have was not necessarily out of difficulty, it was by and large by design. What we were trying to build is a dedicated African sports content wire service because there is a global demand for a lot of African sport like South African rugby, Kenyan distance running, Nigerian table tennis; plenty of demand.

'Media publishers from all over the world can log on to a centralised platform and download video news content, not any different from how an established wire service like AFP or Reuters does it.'

Inspiration was found in the form of an American women's underwear entrepreneur, Sara Blakely according to Stainbank, 'She said if you want to know what your big idea is, write down the five biggest problems you face in a day and one of those problems is your big idea. Just go about sorting it out.

'I love that because access to high quality, up to date sports content is what we all complained about at the time because every media organisation that has some sort of sporting agenda, has a resource problem, with the exception maybe of Sky in Europe, SuperSport in Africa and ESPN and Fox Sports in the U.S.

'That's unfortunate because the majority of interaction with sports content happens with the rest of us. It doesn't happen with pay TV broadcasters or the premium broadcasters. I'm not trying to take anything away from their businesses or how they operate.

'It's silly how good SuperSport is but it still only reaches a third of television viewers on the continent which means there are two-thirds of television viewers on the African continent who are engaging with sports news content that is kind of haphazardly thrown together with what the editors and producers can manage.'

The reality is that at a news channel, there are only so many cameras to go around and news will always take preference over sport. Stainbank says if there are only two cameras available and there are three sports stories taking place at more or less the same time, there is only going to be one outcome.

'You've got Mamelodi Sundowns, Cricket South Africa and netball all at the same time. Who misses out? Netball always misses out and it narrows content so drastically that people can flick channels with their remotes but just see the same thing over and over again.'

Sundowns are one of the most popular football teams in the country and together with the national cricket team, would be commercially more valuable but it is also a self-fulfilling prophecy. If the attitude prevails that Sundowns and the Proteas are more important than netball and therefore always receive coverage preference, then netball will never make any commercial gains and as a by-product struggle to grow as a sport.

The potential is there for coverage of so-called bigger sports like rugby and cricket to suffer from a lack of resources too. Stainbank says the scheduling of the two sports' world cups presents a potential headache to broadcasters, 'The fact that rugby and cricket world cups fall in the same year every single time is a nightmare because the question you effectively have to ask yourself is, "Who might win?"

'Going in, most years, both kind of stand a shot and if you go with the Springboks winning because the Springboks win relatively often, and you decide the Proteas won't win, and then the Proteas do win their first World Cup in their history then you realise, "Oh sh*t, we misdirected our budget entirely" and you're the only media house without a presence at the Cricket World Cup. Then you're done. No one is watching your coverage.'

The vision and intent behind ASCN is to fill gaps but also provide greater access to African sports teams and athletes. Back on the issue of netball, Stainbank says there was a criminal scenario that played out in South Africa, 'Netball South Africa had given SABC free broadcasting rights from 2003 that the SABC just did not bother with.

'It really broke my heart because netball is actually a really, really solid property. In terms of grassroots participation, it's through the charts. It's a solid property that could have been built up over the course of a decade to be so much further than it is now.

'With more relevant content, you can quite quickly turn a weekly 30-minute show which might attract x amount of advertising, into two 30-minute shows a week or one one-hour show a week or whatever the case may be. It's about giving you the opportunity to improve your programming agenda and bring more of that middle tier market of advertisers on board with you because there is a middle tier market of advertisers that can't afford to advertise on SuperSport but they want to be involved in sport.

'The most effective way to do that is to start speaking about short-format news content but in abundance with enough economy of scale so that everybody can have a slice of that pie.'

Stainbank found research time consuming and challenging in the African environment. 'My entire first year was research. I knew that I had an idea for which there was a demand and a need, but it doesn't always translate to a good business.

'If I had the fortune of living in Europe or North America, I might have been able to hop online and maybe with one simple Google search, find out how free-to-air broadcasters and digital media publishers on that continent fair with x and y and z but I don't have that privilege.

'We haven't really started to appreciate data and making data publicly accessible on the African continent. Even when it is available, it tends to be locked away on somebody's hard drive. I had to try to piece it together manually.

I had to figure out what the free-to-air television environment is like in the major markets.

'South Africa was pretty easy to find for most information but Kenya was not so easy to find. I came across so many sites about the Egyptian and Algerian television market that I couldn't find translations for because it was in Arabic,' he says.

Building the business and getting it ready for launch day required hard work, dedication and self-discipline. Stainbank says, 'Despite the fact that I had no employer, no money coming in, I was at my desk at 8 every morning and I checked out at 6 every evening, six days a week.

'Of course, here and there I got a bit distracted and watched a YouTube video but I was at my desk just trying to map out really how big this market is, whether it's justifiable, what the best model might be to accomplish what we're trying to accomplish.

'After that first year, I got to a point in about January of 2019 where I was satisfied with how the business could work, where the price points might be and so forth.'

During this process, Stainbank says he felt "very lonely" because most of his friends of the same age, in and around 30, were getting married, having children, buying houses and cars. Stainbank next made contact with UK-based Gary Rathbone, former SuperSport Head of Africa, who was returning to South Africa. Stainbank set up a coffee meeting and the loneliness almost vanished when Rathbone described ASCN as "the missing link".

'I hadn't had that sort of validation. I'd been alone from 8 to 6 every day, six days a week for a year, so that validation from someone who knew what he was talking about was really, really important to me,' he says.

The pair began working together but found development to be the big stumbling block. Stainbank says, 'I can do editorial all day every day. So can Gary but development was a really tricky thing to find. It was also why we needed some start-up capital.

'I would have liked to have been one of these success stories you hear like, "We had absolutely nothing until we had our first customer", but if I was a developer then maybe, but I'm not and we needed help in that regard.'

At that point, Stainbank was interacting with an investor, but solely for advice. He says, it was someone who he knew personally, 'For about four months, I actually didn't speak to this person about investing in the business. I spoke to him about how he thinks I can get some money.

'I asked if he knew anyone that could invest because it was such an early-stage start-up at that point. It wasn't even a start-up. I wouldn't have even called it a business yet. People would say, "You're running your own business?" and I would say: "Not really." You have people running spaza shops[93] in the hood. They're bringing in money. They're selling a product. That'sa business.'

He knew an angel investor would not give his fledgling "non-business" a second look but that was when this investor offered to get involved, 'When you have been engaging with someone for four, five, six months on your plans, on what you're doing, on the research, they get an inside look into your business and what you're trying to accomplish.

'An angel investor would never have seen that in a 10–15 minute pitch and I had been engaging with this individual for some time, not asking for money but asking how they thought I should progress.'

At some point in that process, he said, 'Look I think you've done really well. Nobody in a 10–15 minute pitch is going to see the underside of the iceberg the way you have been breaking it down to me over the last six months. You're gonna spend an irretrievable amount of time on something that's not gonna get this start-up capital, so I'll be your partner in this.

'I'll come in and give you the money you need for development and the little bits of research that are still outstanding.' Stainbank then had the money he needed.

An important question that lingers in the minds of those considering quitting their jobs to start their own business involves how they will continue to pay the rent or mortgage? How about clothing and feeding the family? What about the children's school fees?

There is a damning statistic that by its very design discourages budding entrepreneurs. Stainbank advises against taking it too seriously, 'I really detest the statistic that is repeated at every conference I go to, every talk I attend, that 80% of new businesses fail.

'It really rubs me up the wrong way because it says absolutely nothing. What happens with a statistic that is as ambiguous as that, is that people can manipulate it to mean whatever they want it to, so if somebody wants to paint a perception

---

[93] A spaza shop is an informal convenience store typically found in a South African township

of young people, or South Africans, as lazy, then they can quote that statistic that 80% of new businesses fail.

'80% of new businesses fail for dozens of reasons but one of them is because people don't have the runway that is required. The financial runway to see the business from inception to profitability and still pay their kids' school fees and that is just an unfortunate and horrible by-product of capitalism, but it doesn't say that people are lazy.

'It doesn't say that people don't know what they're doing. There are so many really smart and capable people that have failed just because the way it is set up is not very easy.'

One of the things that helped Stainbank survive while he was building ASCN was his family. There is a term in Africa known as "black tax". It can loosely be defined as the necessity for young, more educated generations of black people to take care of their parents and grandparents financially.

It tends to set them back in keeping up with their white counterparts. Because of the relatively big size of his family, Stainbank was able to find help, 'We had a lot of financial trouble in my family but we take care of each other. It's not that there's more than enough, but there tends to be enough to go around to just make sure that everyone is okay.

'So for a black person born in the late '80s who went to decent schools to have the education and the foundation that I do and not have to take care of a grandparent or a parent, is a massive advantage that a lot of my peers don't have.

'What it really came down to for me was, what did I stand a chance to lose? I stood a chance to lose the apartment, the car and to a degree, lifestyle but I'm not a very social person. I don't have very expensive tastes in most things. I don't go out a lot. I don't drink. I don't smoke.

'So, those are expenses I don't incur. When it comes to lifestyle for me, coming into this business, if you don't include my apartment, it was groceries, some new clothes now and again, but even then my clothes are from Mr Price[94] typically speaking. I don't do a lot. I don't take extravagant vacations. It wasn't a big loss for me so what I stood to lose was really the apartment and I made peace with that.'

After leaving eNCA, Stainbank still made an initial attempt at some income while building ASCN, 'I thought that what I was going to do was make this web

---

[94] Mr Price is a budget clothing and accessories store catering to lower-middle and middle-income consumers

series happen and then I was going to build ASCN at the same time and it didn't take place that way but by the time I stopped working on the web series and realised it was taking up more of my time and resources and energy than is justifiable, I had by that point reached a point with ASCN where I couldn't fit in anything else.

'I was working solid full days, so people would say to me, "Why don't you write?" just to bring in a bit of money, and they were right, but I was actually working on ASCN so much around the clock that I didn't think that I could really sit down and apply myself the way I would like to apply myself to freelance writing.

'When that realisation occurred to me, I knew the web series I tried to produce wasn't going to work out and I knew ASCN was still a really long way away. I still had that two-and-a-half year goal and I realised that I was submerging myself so much in ASCN that I really didn't have the mental capacity or the time to work on anything else, so I said okay, the apartment is going to have to go.'

Losing his apartment was something that he accepted as a possibility and fortunately, there was alternative accommodation nearby, 'I didn't have to move to another city to move back in with my parents. My mother actually lives in Bloemfontein where she works, and my brother stays in her house (in Johannesburg) so I moved in with my brother.'

Living in his mother's house drastically helped cut Stainbank's monthly expenses. He had some savings that he mostly used to maintain his car instalments but despite his best frugal intentions, one year after leaving his job, he was out of money.

That set the stage for this heart-warming story Stainbank shares, 'My grandmother was going on a cruise in early 2019 and I was supposed to take her to the airport. She came to my mother's house. There's a bunch of people in the house and I'm in the kitchen fetching glasses because I'm going to pour everyone some juice and my grandmother corners me in the kitchen and closes the door.

'She inquires, "How much money do you have?" I thought she needed me to run to the store. I might have had twenty bucks and she inquired again, "No, no. How much money do you have left?"

I said, "I'm nearly out".

She asked, "What do you mean, nearly out?"

I said, "After I pay my next car instalment, I've got no money".

'She said, "Okay, you direct those debits to my account. Don't tell anybody". That was February of 2019 and my grandmother died in August. During that period, she paid four car instalments for me and then I got the investment that I needed.

'She paid four months for me and the month that she died, August 2019, was the month I was going to say to her, "You can stop paying". I was the most excited person in the world to tell her, "Thank you for the last few months but I got this investment. I'm gonna take a small stipend and I'll be able to pay for my car going forward", and then she passed away before I could tell her that. It still breaks my heart. I can't say enough about that sacrifice and how grateful I am for it.'

ASCN successfully launched in September 2020 and no doubt, there would not have been a person on Earth prouder than Mrs Kamo Smith. This chapter is dedicated to her memory.

Chapter Fourteen
The Future

The most appropriate way to complete this book is to attempt to give a glance into what the future may hold. Soothsaying or clairvoyance is however futile. There is no reliably accurate crystal ball. I remember as a 15-year-old boy listening to the radio in the wee hours on 5 July 1999.

The presenter announced that Nostradamus had predicted that this was to be the day on which the world would end. I broke out in a cold sweat. My birthday is the 12th of July! How could the world end just one week before my birthday? I thought that tremendously unfair.

Moreover, a friend of mine told me in 2006 that Spain would win the FIFA World Cup to be held in Germany. His source was the same Nostradamus who, according to my friend, had predicted that in 2006, the Spanish forces would cross the Pyrenees, defeat the evil forces and return with the Holy Grail.

Well, Italy won that year's World Cup. I have never bothered to verify any of those predictions, but it is curious how Spain was going to go about this mission in the first place given that the world would have supposedly ended seven years earlier.

Sports betting is another attempt at trying to see into the future. You will recall the story I shared with you from 2009 where I lost a lot of money betting on the top-of-the-table Sharks against the winless bottom-of-the-standings Cheetahs in a Super Rugby match. The Cheetahs won so comfortably you would have thought it was the Sharks who were without a victory up to that point.

So instead of making wild predictions, let us instead look at the state of journalism as it stands today, consider the changing nature of the modern newsroom, and look at how best modern journalists can equip themselves for a future that is as exciting as it is uncertain.

It seems as if I hear about newsroom downscaling or journalism redundancies on a weekly basis. It is scary, make no mistake. In May 2020, Microsoft announced it was replacing around 50 journalists with automated technology on its MSN website. According to Microsoft, it was part of an evaluation of its business.

A Microsoft staffer told *The Seattle Times*, 'It's demoralising to think machines can replace us but there you go.'[95] Wherever you work, at some stage you can expect "an evaluation of business" and you, or someone you know, is likely to be on the chopping block. You can do whatever you can to make yourself indispensable, but the reality is that it will not matter much to the accountants.

It remains to be seen how well artificial intelligence handles strict editorial guidelines. Google has already made available artificial intelligence to the point where you could have your very own Google personal assistant answering or making telephone calls and appointments on your behalf. It is called Google Duplex. [96]

Google has since been forced into competing with the highly successful ChatGPT AI service which has caused major disruptions since its launch in late 2022.

It is an uncertain time in journalism. Some of the developments are exciting while others make many people feel uneasy. It is fair to say journalists are being asked to do more and often without the appropriate compensation. Understandably, staff are disgruntled.

This is not just applicable to sports journalism. Take Bari Weiss for example. She published her resignation letter from *The New York Times* online to bring attention to the conditions she experienced at the famed newspaper. Weiss wrote, 'I was hired with the goal of bringing in voices that would not otherwise appear in your pages: first-time writers, centrists, conservatives and others who would not naturally think of The Times as their home.

---

[95] The Seattle Times. (2020). Microsoft is cutting dozens of MSN news production workers and replacing them with artificial intelligence. [online] Available at: https://www.seattletimes.com/business/local-business/microsoft-is-cutting-dozens-of-msn-news-production-workers-and-replacing-them-with-artificial-intelligence/.

[96] Google Duplex: A.I. Assistant Calls Local Businesses To Make Appointments. (2018). YouTube. Available at: https://www.youtube.com/watch?v=D5VN56jQMWM.

'The reason for this effort was clear: The paper's failure to anticipate the outcome of the 2016 (U.S. presidential) election meant that it didn't have a firm grasp of the country it covers.'

In the letter, she mentioned the diverse list of names she brought to the pages of the famous newspaper but then lamented how the warnings from 2016 had not been heeded, 'The lessons that ought to have followed the election—lessons about the importance of understanding other Americans, the necessity of resisting tribalism, and the centrality of the free exchange of ideas to a democratic society—have not been learned.

'Instead, a new consensus has emerged in the press, but perhaps especially at this paper: that truth isn't a process of collective discovery, but an orthodoxy already known to an enlightened few whose job is to inform everyone else.'

She went on to write about the influence of social media and what she views as news targeted at a small audience only, 'Twitter is not on the masthead of *The New York Times*. But Twitter has become its ultimate editor. As the ethics and mores of that platform have become those of the paper, the paper itself has increasingly become a kind of performance space.

'Stories are chosen and told in a way to satisfy the narrowest of audiences, rather than to allow a curious public to read about the world and then draw their own conclusions. I was always taught that journalists were charged with writing the first rough draft of history.

'Now, history itself is one more ephemeral thing moulded to fit the needs of a predetermined narrative.'

'In this letter, Weiss shared how she even experienced intimidation in the workplace for not toeing the line: *My own forays into Wrongthink have made me the subject of constant bullying by colleagues who disagree with my views. They have called me a Nazi and a racist; I have learnt to brush off comments about how I'm "writing about the Jews again".*

'Several colleagues perceived to be friendly with me were badgered by co-workers. My work and my character are openly demeaned on company-wide Slack channels where masthead editors regularly weigh in. There, some co-workers insist I need to be rooted out if this company is to be a truly "inclusive" one, while others post axe emojis next to my name.

'Still other New York Times employees publicly smear me as a liar and a bigot on Twitter with no fear that harassing me will be met with appropriate action. They never are. There are terms for all of this: unlawful discrimination, hostile work environment, and constructive discharge.

'I'm no legal expert. But I know that this is wrong. I do not understand how you have allowed this kind of behaviour to go on inside your company in full view of the paper's entire staff and the public. And I certainly can't square how you and other Times leaders have stood by while simultaneously praising me in private for my courage.

'Showing up for work as a centrist at an American newspaper should not require bravery. Part of me wishes I could say that my experience was unique. But the truth is that intellectual curiosity – let alone risk-taking – is now a liability at The Times.

'Why edit something challenging to our readers, or write something bold only to go through the numbing process of making it ideologically kosher, when we can assure ourselves of job security (and clicks) by publishing our 4000th op-ed arguing that Donald Trump is a unique danger to the country and the world? And so self-censorship has become the norm.

'What rules that remain at The Times are applied with extreme selectivity. If a person's ideology is in keeping with the new orthodoxy, they and their work remain unscrutinised. Everyone else lives in fear of the digital thunder dome.

'Online venom is excused so long as it is directed at the proper targets. Op-eds that would have easily been published just two years ago would now get an editor or a writer in serious trouble, if not fired. If a piece is perceived as likely to inspire backlash internally or on social media, the editor or writer avoids pitching it.'[97]

While Weiss' situation is mostly of a socio-political ideological nature, do not think that sport escapes this kind of treatment. Remember what you read earlier about the Irish journalist David Walsh who first exposed Lance Armstrong's doping at the Tour de France?

Walsh was vilified by Armstrong and his handlers, as expected, but was also unpopular with many of his media colleagues; many of whom were happy to simply cheerlead for the American cyclist. It took more than a decade for Armstrong to finally admit to doping. I wonder how many reporters and editors issued Walsh with a much-deserved apology.

---

[97] Bari Weiss. (n.d.). Resignation Letter. [online] Available at: https://www.bariweiss.com/resignation-letter.

Matti Taibbi published a piece on his website entitled *The American Press Is Destroying Itself.* Taibbi cites *The New York Times* editorial page editor, James Bennet who was ousted for approving an anti-protest editorial by Tom Cotton, an Arkansas Republican senator.

Cotton's piece was published in the aftermath of the heinous killing of George Floyd, a black man, at the hands of a white police officer. The killing sparked widespread protests across the United States. In an apology, Marc Tracy wrote, 'James Bennet, the editorial page editor of *The New York Times*, has resigned after a controversy over an op-ed by a senator calling for military force against protesters in American cities.'

That was changed to: 'James Bennet resigned on Sunday from his job as the editorial page editor of *The New York Times*, days after the newspaper's opinion section, which he oversaw, published a much-criticised op-ed by a United States senator calling for a military response to civic unrest in American cities.'

As Taibbi stressed, 'Cotton did not call for "military force against protesters in American cities". He spoke of a "show of force", to rectify a situation a significant portion of the country saw as spiralling out of control. It's an important distinction.

'Cotton was presenting one side of the most important question on the most important issue of a critically important day in American history. As Cotton points out in the piece, he was advancing a view arguably held by a majority of the country.

'A *Morning Consult* poll showed 58% of Americans either strongly or somewhat supported the idea of "calling in the U.S. military to supplement city police forces". That survey included 40% of self-described "liberals" and 37% of African-Americans.

'To declare a point of view held by that many people not only not worthy of discussion, but so toxic that publication of it without even necessarily agreeing requires dismissal, is a dramatic reversal for a newspaper that long cast itself as the national paper of record.'[98]

Regardless of your personal view on racism, police brutality and protests, you can appreciate how the above scenarios can make for uncomfortable

---

[98] Taibbi, M. (2020). The American Press Is Destroying Itself. [online] TK News by Matt Taibbi. Available at: https://taibbi.substack.com/p/the-news-media-is-destroying-itself [Accessed 6 June 2020].

conversations and even conflicting ethical conundrums for reporters in the newsroom.

The easiest way to escape that kind of toxicity is to work for yourself in a freelance or entrepreneurial capacity. Easier said than done of course but in the modern environment, it would be worth your while to at least have a blog, podcast or YouTube channel as a side hustle.

If you do go that route, it is crucial you hold yourself to the highest journalistic standards and ethics. In this instance, you can again see how important it is to be multi-skilled.

Sport remains one of the few remaining content types where fans will go out of their way to watch it live. After all, the FIFA World Cup final is not Season 10 of *The Big Bang Theory*. That said there are ever-changing ways to keep those same fans engaged.

According to Deloitte[99], sports fans spend up to three times more than casual fans on streaming, and 1.5 times more than casual fans on broadcast. Sports streaming remains a social experience, though the desired experience depends heavily on demographics and the sport in question.

A Deloitte sports fan survey shows that overall satisfaction is only 39% for the broadcast and OTT experience, leaving significant opportunity for continued technological advancement for fans looking to consume sports across devices and integrate augmented reality (AR), virtual reality (VR), social media, and gambling into their viewing experience.

Before we continue, let us establish a few definitions:

OTT – Over The Top. A reference to content delivered via an internet connection rather than through a traditional cable/satellite service.

Augmented Reality – An interactive experience where your real-world environment is enhanced by incorporating computer-generated objects and information.

Virtual Reality – Computer-generated simulation of a three-dimensional image or environment that can be interacted with in a seemingly real or physical way by a person using special electronic equipment, such as a helmet with a screen inside or gloves fitted with sensors.

---

[99] Deloitte United States. (2019). Enhancing Digital Fan Engagement. [online] Available at: https://www2.deloitte.com/us/en/pages/technology-media-and-telecommunications/articles/enhancing-digital-fan-engagement.html.

Personally, I like the concept of augmented reality a lot more than virtual reality. The thought of thousands of people walking around dressed in computer-powered helmets resembling Power Rangers is not one that excites me, and yet, more than 54% of fans surveyed by Deloitte, indicated that virtual reality front-row seats would increase their likelihood to watch a game.

The Deloitte report argues that sport is important in driving viewership for channels, and this in turn can drive spending. Big sports fans are more than twice as likely as casual fans to spend on sports-related OTT streaming and broadcast.

Among those fans who spend on subscriptions, the biggest fans spend approximately 1.5 times more than casual fans on cable subscription but among Millennials (generally people born between 1981 and 1996) and Generation Z (generally people born between 1997 and 2012), the biggest fans spend nearly three times more than casual fans on streaming services to watch sport.

With that in mind, you can see why Spotify would spend hundreds of millions of dollars acquiring podcasts like *The Ringer*. The emergence of ESPN+, DAZN and Hulu begins to make a lot of sense too.

Many things are changing in sport and journalism, but as long as there is a zealous appetite for live sport there will be a market for news. This is great news for a young sports journalist concerned about doomsday prophecies predicting an imminent death for journalism.

As this book is being written, 5G is in the early stages of global rollout. This is going to make for a massive improvement in wireless connectivity and create all kinds of possibilities in the digital landscape. As a journalist, you want to make it your business to stay up to date and see what you can incorporate into your personal toolbox.

What does this mean for sport? Nielsen Sports global marketing director Glenn Lovett says it means opportunity, 'Barriers to entry have never been lower. More markets around the world than ever before are receptive to the power of sports. It's never been easier to reach millions, even billions, of fans.' Lovett could just as well be speaking to you and every other sports journalist out there.

It is important to emphasise that not everything new will be worth your while but look into it anyway. Perhaps you might find a way to use a piece of equipment or software to enhance your output. I started out as a radio presenter. My only real skill was talking in between songs.

Now, I am capable of television presenting, reporting, script writing, voicing, podcasting, camera operating and video editing. Admittedly, the last two skills are a work in progress, but I am better than I was a year ago, and a year ago I was better than I was a year before that. Oh, and it would seem as if book-writing is also a part of my skill set now!

It is worth remembering that even if the traditional television viewing model for sport is disrupted, that does not mean there is no place for journalism in sport. Assume sport is no longer on the television, you can be sure that Gianni Infantino will make sure the FIFA World Cup is accessible to the masses in another way. Perhaps the only way for millions of people to watch the tournament in the future will be to dress up as a Power Ranger!

What you can be certain of, is that as long as there is a FIFA, an IOC, an ANOC and so forth, there will be a need for sports journalism. The bad guys will not go away just because consumer habits have changed.

In terms of broadcast rights, there is a hint that the likes of Facebook, Amazon and others are looking to develop sustainable business models to gobble up sports rights. Who is to say how this might play out? Again, be mindful of it and try to position yourself in such a way that you are ready for it.

It could be that there is a daily sports news bulletin on Facebook. Perhaps Facebook will begin to air sports-specific documentaries, the likes of which have already been seen on Netflix and Amazon Prime for example. That will require producers, presenters, cameramen, researchers, writers, video editors and so on. Be ready.

Nielsen predicted that sports that cannot demonstrate their social usefulness will lose business to those that can.[100] That was an interesting observation but as a journalist, you want to be equally, if not more, mindful of the sports that are appearing to be socially useful.

Think of social justice, equality, racism, sexism and so forth, then hold the federation, administrators, or athletes accountable. Are they really trying to make a difference or is it just lip service? There is a story there for a journalist.

Nielsen has also found that Generation Z prefers faster-paced sports. In their report *Game Changer: Rethinking Sports Experiences For Generation Z,* they

---

[100] TOP 5 GLOBAL SPORTS INDUSTRY TRENDS 2. (n.d.). [online] Available at: http://nielsensports.com/wp-content/uploads/2014/09/nielsen-top-5-commercial-sports-trends-2018.pdf.

found this younger demographic likes basketball, extreme sports, mixed martial arts, surfing and field hockey more than their older counterparts on average.

Similarly, they like baseball, motorsport and golf less than those in older demographics. Motorsport and field hockey appear to me at least to be in contradictory places but who am I to question the tastes of other people? My favourite sports are cricket, tennis, rugby, football and boxing.

The latter two are traditionally associated with the working class while the other three range from middle class to private school elitism. Talk about a contradiction!

Those are issues that the individual sports will have to grapple with. However, it should provide you with an insight into the changing likes and dislikes of the various demographics. If you have read that and come away with the thought that becoming a niche journalist covering the Ultimate Fighting Championship or World Surf League, then go for it.

It is impossible to predict what will happen next in terms of sports journalism. Yes, we know that robots are replacing us in some instances. Yes, technology is changing all the time and we are forced to adapt at every turn. There are many reporters who never imagined when they were starting out in the late 1990s that one day they would have to take their own camera and tripod to press conferences but that is increasingly the norm.

The best advice I can dispense is to embrace the change and have as many skills and abilities in your toolbox as you possibly can. The reality is that for most of us, no company will deem us indispensable but by being multi-skilled, you position yourself favourably.

The company might be less likely to make you redundant because you bring more to the table. Further to that, it might be easier for you to land a new job in a shorter space of time because of your varied skill set. A multi-skilled operator is also better positioned to achieve success as a freelancer or in entrepreneurship. A one-trick pony is likely to be left in the stable while the other thoroughbreds run the race.

Co-founder of *Seen*, Yusuf Omar foresees journalists playing a different role in the future, 'By 2030, we believe that everyone will be wearing camera glasses on their faces and that your computer experience will move from a phone, or a computer, or iPad, to a computer that's on your face.

'I think that all journalists need to be ready for that future in terms of building augmented reality experiences so that people can experience their journalism on whichever surface they want. I think that increasingly people are going to be the first boots on the ground for major stories.

'Social media platforms will provide you with the "what happened, where it happened and when it happened". I think journalists are going to focus on "the why and the how" and I think they're gonna play a god's eye view on the world looking at billions of mobile videos and trying to work out what's real and what isn't.

'I think the role of the journalist is going to move from the creator to the curator and I think that the core responsibilities are going to move to fact checking and verifying and trying to identify the voices among all of the noise.'

Journalism and technology collided a long time ago and the relationship will only grow stronger. Omar adds, 'I think the intersection between journalism and being a technologist is really important. Understanding how people can consume today is fine, but I think you need to be preparing for how they will consume tomorrow.'

In conclusion, let me say that you do not need to be fearful of this industry or its future. Yes, it is tough and there are difficult people, sometimes downright nasty and mean-spirited individuals, and challenging circumstances, but ultimately the rewards comfortably outweigh the negatives.

What a wonderful privilege it is to be able to watch live sport and cover athletes for a living. Of course, there is so much more to it than that but ultimately, you will be doing a job that millions of people dream they could be doing.

No one sits at their desk thinking, "I should have become a toll booth operator". Embrace the madness, upskill yourself at every opportunity, hold those you cover accountable, hold yourself accountable to the highest journalistic ethics and enjoy every moment of it. That is how you become a sports journalist.

References

Chapter Two

1. www.dictionary.com. (n.d.). Definition of journalism | Dictionary.com. [online] Available at: https://www.dictionary.com/browse/journalism?s=t.
2. American Press Institute (2019). What is journalism? Definition and meaning of the craft. [online] American Press Institute. Available at: https://www.americanpressinstitute.org/journalism-essentials/what-is-journalism/.
3. Wikipedia Contributors (2019). Journalism. [online] Wikipedia. Available at: https://en.wikipedia.org/wiki/Journalism.
4. Jennings, A. (2016) *The dirty game: uncovering the scandal at FIFA,* London: Arrow Books. (pp 120–121)
5. Hartley, R. (2016) *The big fix: how South Africa stole the World Cup,* Johannesburg: Jonathan Ball Publishers. (pp 38 67)
6. Jennings, A. (2016) *The dirty game: uncovering the scandal at FIFA,* London: Arrow Books. (p 113)
7. Sky Sports. (n.d.). Ex-FIFA chief Jack Warner in UK court appeal against corruption charges. [online] Available at: https://www.skysports.com/football/news/11095/11978212/ex-fifa-chief-jack-warner-in-uk-court-appeal-against-corruption-charges) [Accessed on 23 May 2020].
8. Vyv Simson and Jennings, A. (1992) *The lords of the rings: power, money and drugs in the modern Olympics,* London: Simon & Schuster.
9. Joffe, G. (2019) *Sport: greed & betrayal.* Independently Published. p 251
10. Joffe, G. (2019) *Sport: greed & betrayal.* Independently Published. p 259

11. Joffe, G. (2019) *Sport: greed & betrayal.* Independently Published. p 251

12. Joffe, G. (2019) *Sport: greed & betrayal.* Independently Published. pp 86–87

13. Joffe, G. (2019) *Sport: greed & betrayal.* Independently Published. p 200

14. Joffe, G. (2019) *Sport: greed & betrayal.* Independently Published. p 36

15. Joffe, G. (2019) *Sport: greed & betrayal.* Independently Published. pp 196–205

16. ESPNcricinfo. (n.d.). Mohammad Amir profile and biography, stats, records, averages, photos and videos. [online] Available at: https://www.espncricinfo.com/pakistan/content/player/290948.html [Accessed 23 May 2020].

17. ESPNcricinfo. (n.d.). Hansie Cronje profile and biography, stats, records, averages, photos and videos. [online] Available at: https://www.espncricinfo.com/southafrica/content/player/44485.html [Accessed 23 May 2020].

18. Published, C.S. (2021). Lance Armstrong | Cycling Weekly. [online] cyclingweekly.com. Available at: https://www.cyclingweekly.com/tag/lance-armstrong [Accessed 23 May 2020].

19. The Guardian. (2014). How I brought down drug-taking Lance Armstrong, by David Walsh. [online] Available at: https://www.theguardian.com/media/greenslade/2014/jan/28/lance-armstrong-sundaytimes.

20. Kroeger, B. and Hamill, P. (2012). CRUSADERS AND ZEALOTS. [online] JSTOR. Available at: http://www.jstor.org/stable/j.ctt22727sf.16 [Accessed 24 May 2020]. (pp. 209–210)

21. QARA (2019). Sports Industry Insights. [online] Medium. Available at: https://medium.com/qara/sports-industry-report-3244bd253b8.

22. FUTURE OF GLOBAL SPORT ASSOCIATION OF SUMMER OLYMPIC INTERNATIONAL FEDERATIONS. (2019). [online] Available at: https://www.asoif.com/sites/default/files/download/future_of_global_sport.pdf.

23. Anon, (n.d.). [online] Available at: http://www.measure4you.de/images/AnalysisOfOnlineMarketingInThe Spo rtsIndustry.pdf.

24. Fosket, S. (1996, November) 'Online technology ushers in one-to-one market,' *Direct Marketing,* 59, 7, 38–40

25. Shandu, K. (2008, February/March) 'The Business of Soccer and Television-What's In It?,' *Journal of Marketing*, pp 65–79

26. DCMS (2009). Review of Free-to-air Listed Events Report by the Independent Advisory Panel to the Secretary of State for Culture, Media and Sport. [online] Available at: http://webarchive.nationalarchives.gov.uk/+/http:/www.culture.gov.uk/i ma ges/consultations/independentpanelreport-to-SoS-Free-to-air-Nov2009.pdf [Accessed 4 November 2018].

27. Gemmell, J. (2018) 'BBC Sport in Black and White, by Richard Haynes,' *The International Journal of the History of Sport,* 35, 11, pp 1209–1211.

28. Deloitte (2021). Deloitte Football Money League | Deloitte UK. [online] Deloitte United Kingdom. Available at: https://www2.deloitte.com/uk/en/pages/sports-business-group/articles/deloitte-football-money-league.html.

29. https://www2.deloitte.com/content/dam/Deloitte/uk/Documents/sports-business-group/deloitte-uk-annual-review-of-football-finance-2019.pdf (Michael Barnard, Sam Boor, Christopher Winn, Chris Wood and Izzy Wray)

30. Ronal do Economi cs. (n.d.). [online] Available at: https://www.footballbenchmark.com/documents/files/public/KPMG%2 0Foo tball%20Benchmark_Ronaldo%20Economics(1).pdf.

31. Anon, (n.d.). Messi's Departure Could Cost Barcelona €137 Million in Brand Value | Press Release | Brand Finance. [online] Available at: https://brandfinance.com/press-releases/messi-departure-could-cost-barcelona-137-million-in-brand-value.

32. http://nielsensports.com/wp-content/uploads/2014/09/FIFAReport-2018.pdf.

33. QARA (2019). Sports Industry Insights. [online] Medium. Available at: https://medium.com/qara/sports-industry-report-3244bd253b8.

34. Durent, J. (n.d.). Kevin McNaughton reveals shock and sympathy at Wigan Athletic plight as club highlights financial and ownership shortcomings of Championship life. [online] Press and Journal. Available at: https://www.pressandjournal.co.uk/fp/sport/football/2327207/2327207/ [Accessed 25 May 2020].

35. South China Morning Post. (2020). Finger-pointing, the Philippines and EFL-what happened at Wigan? [online] Available at: https://www.scmp.com/sport/football/article/3092949/wigan-athletic-and-hong-kong-based-mystery-finger-pointing [Accessed 25 May 2020].

36. Giorgio, P. (2019). Deloitte's sports industry trends for 2019. [online] Deloitte United States. Available at: https://www2.deloitte.com/us/en/pages/technology-media-and-telecommunications/articles/sports-business-trends-disruption.html.

37. Gillett, A.G. (2017) 'The business of sports agents,' *Business History,* 61, 2, pp 374–375.

38. Deloitte United Kingdom. (n.d.). Falcon and Associates/Dubai Sports Council-Economic Impact of Sport in Dubai. [online] Available at: https://www2.deloitte.com/uk/en/pages/sports-business-group/articles/economic-impact-of-sport-in-dubai.html [Accessed 22 May 2020].

39. ITTF Strategic Plan. (2018). [online] Available at: https://www.ittf.com/wp-content/uploads/2018/08/ITTF-Strategic-Plan-en.pdf.

40. Anon, (n.d.). [online] Available at: http://www.measure4you.de/images/AnalysisOfOnlineMarketingInThe Spo rtsIndustry.pdf.

41. Press, A.A. (2019) 'Rugby's LeBron James': Toronto confirm Sonny Bill Williams signing. [online] the Guardian. Available at: https://www.theguardian.com/sport/2019/nov/08/rugbys-lebron-james-toronto-confirm-sonny-bill-williams-signing [Accessed 26 May 2020].

42. FUTURE OF GLOBAL SPORT ASSOCIATION OF SUMMER OLYMPIC INTERNATIONAL FEDERATIONS. (2019). [online] Available at:

https://www.asoif.com/sites/default/files/download/future_of_global_sp ort.pdf.

43. Evens, T., Petros Iosifidis and Smith, P. (2013) *The political economy of television sports rights,* Basingstoke, Palgrave Macmillan.

44. Boardman, A.E. and Hargreaves-Heap, S.P. (1999) *Journal of Cultural Economics,* 23, 3, pp 165–179.

45. Scherer, J. and Sam, M.P. (2012) 'Public Broadcasting, Sport and Cultural Citizenship: Sky's the Limit in New Zealand,' *Media Culture & Society,* 34, 10, pp 101–111

46. Musa, M. (2014) *Sport, Public Broadcasting, and Cultural Citizenship: Signal Lost?* Location: ROUTLEDGE.

47. Sullivan, G. (2009) *Television and the 2006 World Cup: National Narrative of Pride and Party Patriotism,* Germany.

48. Castello, E., Dhoest, A. and O'Donnell, H. (eds.) *The Nation on Screen, Discourses of the National in Global Television,* Cambridge: Cambridge Scholars Press.

49. Evens, T., Petros Iosifidis and Smith, P. (2013) *The political economy of television sports rights,* Basingstoke, Palgrave Macmillan.

Chapter Three

1. newspaper | History & Facts. (2019). In: Encyclopædia Britannica. [online] Available at: https://www.britannica.com/topic/newspaper.

2. The Guardian. (2020). Mehdi Hasan: 'Most people ask the question and move on. I don't.' [online] Available at: https://www.theguardian.com/tv-and-radio/2020/mar/27/mehdi-hasan-interview [Accessed 27 May 2020].

3. Coleman, R., McCombs, M., Shaw, D. and Weaver, D. (2009) *The Handbook of Journalism Studies* [e-book] New York: Routledge. Available through: Edinburgh Napier University Library website.

4. <https://ebookcentral.proquest.com/lib/napier/reader.action?docID=40 1841 &query=> [Accessed 19 September 2018].

5. Weaver, D. (1991) 'Issue salience and public opinion: Are there consequences of agenda-setting?' *International Journal of Public Opinion*, 3, pp 53–68.

Chapter Four

1. Wikipedia. (2022). Debora Patta. [online] Available at: https://en.wikipedia.org/wiki/Debora_Patta [Accessed 28 May 2020].
2. The Guardian. (2020). Mehdi Hasan: 'Most people ask the question and move on. I don't.' [online] Available at: https://www.theguardian.com/tv-and-radio/2020/mar/27/mehdi-hasan-interview.
3. Avant, D. (n.d.). On how Mehdi Hasan caught Erik Prince in a lie. [online] www.aljazeera.com. Available at: https://www.aljazeera.com/indepth/opinion/mehdi-hasan-caught-erik-prince-lie-190315125456331.html [Accessed 28 May 2020].

Chapter Five

1. newspaper | History & Facts. (2019). In: Encyclopædia Britannica. [online] Available at: https://www.britannica.com/topic/newspaper.
2. The Athletic. (2019). The Athletic. [online] Available at: https://theathletic.com/.
3. Berger, J. (2014) *Contagious: how to build word of mouth in the digital age,* London: Simon & Schuster. pp 22–25
4. Berger, J. (2014) *Contagious: how to build word of mouth in the digital age,* London: Simon & Schuster. p 109
5. Federal Communications Commission. (2017). What We Do. [online] Available at: https://www.fcc.gov/about-fcc/what-we-do.
6. The Independent. (2019). Gary Lineker volunteers to cut down £1.75m BBC salary. [online] Available at: https://www.independent.co.uk/arts-entertainment/tv/news/gary-lineker-bbc-salary-match-of-the-day-a9108286.html [Accessed 29 May 2020].
7. Forbes. (n.d.). Bill Simmons. [online] Available at: https://www.forbes.com/profile/bill-simmons/#1ada4e7648ce [Accessed 29 May 2020].
8. Shapiro, A. (n.d.). Spotify Sale Mints The Ringer's Bill Simmons As Podcasting's First Big-Money Superstar. [online] Forbes. Available at: https://www.forbes.com/sites/arielshapiro/2020/06/04/spotify-sale-

mints-the-ringers-bill-simmons-as-podcastings-first-big-money-superstar/#23fa7e837e52 [Accessed 29 May 2020].

9. TechCrunch. (n.d.). Spotify is buying The Ringer to boost its sports podcast content. [online] Available at: https://techcrunch.com/2020/02/05/spotify-is-buying-the-ringer-to-boost-its-sports-podcast-content/ [Accessed 29 May 2020].

10. Dude Perfect Wiki. (n.d.). Cory. [online] Available at: https://dudeperfect.fandom.com/wiki/Cory_Cotton [Accessed 5 May 2022].

11. Dude Perfect. (2019). YouTube. Available at: https://www.youtube.com/user/corycotton.

Chapter Six

1. Times Higher Education (THE). (2021). World University Rankings. [online] Available at: https://www.timeshighereducation.com/world-university-rankings/2022/world-ranking#.

2. Dean of Undergraduate Students. (n.d.). Core Curriculum for Undergraduates. [online] Available at: https://www.deans.caltech.edu/core-curriculum-undergraduates [Accessed 30 May 2020].

3. Napier. (n.d.). Courses. [online] Available at: https://www.napier.ac.uk/courses?q=journalism [Accessed 30 May 2020].

4. www.humanities.uct.ac.za. (n.d.). Degrees & programmes | Faculty of Humanities. [online] Available at: http://www.humanities.uct.ac.za/hum/undergraduate/degrees.

5. Explore your options for 2018. (n.d.). [online] Available at: http://www.humanities.uct.ac.za/sites/default/files/image_tool/images/2/20 18%20UGHum%20EXplo%20web.pdf [Accessed 30 May 2020].

6. Top Universities. (n.d.). Journalism Degrees. [online] Available at: https://www.topuniversities.com/courses/journalism/guide [Accessed 6 May 2022].

7. www.collegefactual.com. (n.d.). 2022 Best Journalism Bachelor's Degree Schools. [online] Available at: https://www.collegefactual.com/majors/communication-journalism-

media/journalism/rankings/top-ranked/bachelors-degrees/ [Accessed 6 May 2022].

8. The Best Journalism Schools (2013). The Best Journalism Schools. [online] College Factual. Available at: https://www.collegefactual.com/majors/communication-journalism-media/journalism/rankings/top-ranked/.

9. The Open University. (n.d.). R14 | BA (Hons) Arts and Humanities (Creative Writing). [online] Available at: http://www.openuniversity.edu/courses/qualifications/r14-cw [Accessed 30 May 2020].

Chapter Seven

1. www.bestlawyers.com. (n.d.). Best Sports Lawyers in Canada. [online] Available at: https://www.bestlawyers.com/canada/sports-law [Accessed 31 May 2020].

2. United States Courts. (n.d.). New York Times v. Sullivan Podcast. [online] Available at: https://www.uscourts.gov/about-federal-courts/educational-resources/supreme-court-landmarks/new-york-times-v-sullivan-podcast.

3. www.ncsl.org. (2008). At-Will Employment-Overview. [online] Available at: https://www.ncsl.org/research/labor-and-employment/at-will-employment-overview.aspx#:~:text=At%2Dwill%20means%20that%20an.

Chapter Eight

1. Andrea Koppel (2019). How to Break Into Journalism, Even If It Wasn't Your Major. [online] Time4Coffee. Available at: https://time4coffee.org/how-to-break-into-journalism-even-if-it-wasnt-your-major/ [Accessed 31 May 2020].

2. Andrea Koppel (2019). How to Break Into Journalism, Even If It Wasn't Your Major. [online] Time4Coffee. Available at: https://time4coffee.org/how-to-break-into-journalism-even-if-it-wasnt-your-major/.

Chapter Nine

1. BestColleges.com. (2019). Journalism Careers | BestColleges. [online] Available at: https://www.bestcolleges.com/careers/humanities-and-social-sciences/journalism/.
2. Encyclopaedia Britannica. (n.d.). Shorthand. [online] Available at: https://www.britannica.com/topic/shorthand.
3. Hollier, D. (2014). How to Write 225 Words Per Minute With a Pen. [online] The Atlantic. Available at: https://www.theatlantic.com/technology/archive/2014/06/yeah-i-still-use-shorthand-and-a-smartpen/373281/ [Accessed 1 June 2020].

Chapter Ten

1. Gungor, M. (2017) 'Discovering your heart with the Flag Page: a simple and powerful way to truly understand yourself and others,' *Laugh Your Way America!* Lyc. p 17.
2. Gungor, M. (2017) 'Discovering your heart with the Flag Page: a simple and powerful way to truly understand yourself and others,' *Laugh Your Way America!* Llc. p 19.
3. Gungor, M. (2017) 'Discovering your heart with the Flag Page: a simple and powerful way to truly understand yourself and others,' *Laugh Your Way America!* Llc. p 21–22
4. Gungor, M. (2017) 'Discovering your heart with the Flag Page: a simple and powerful way to truly understand yourself and others,' *Laugh Your Way America!* Llc. p 27–44

Chapter Eleven

1. www.dictionary.com. (n.d.). Definition of journalism | Dictionary.com. [online] Available at: https://www.dictionary.com/browse/journalism?s=t.

2. South Africanism. The best possible English translation is "point and shoot". It usually describes a cheaper, less advanced camera designed for only the basics.
3. Afrikaanse Hoër Seunskool. A famous boys-only high school in Pretoria.

Chapter Twelve

1. The Seattle Times. (2020). Microsoft is cutting dozens of MSN news production workers and replacing them with artificial intelligence. [online] Available at: https://www.seattletimes.com/business/local-business/microsoft-is-cutting-dozens-of-msn-news-production-workers-and-replacing-them-with-artificial-intelligence/.
2. Twitter. (n.d.). https://twitter.com/hwalker_brown/status/1276453109313740807. [online] Available at: https://twitter.com/HWalker_Brown/status/1276453109313740807 [Accessed 4 June 2020].

Chapter Thirteen

1. A spaza shop is an informal convenience store typically found in a South African township.
2. Mr Price is a budget clothing and accessories store catering to lower-middle and middle-income consumers.

Chapter Fourteen

1. The Seattle Times. (2020). Microsoft is cutting dozens of MSN news production workers and replacing them with artificial intelligence. [online] Available at: https://www.seattletimes.com/business/local-business/microsoft-is-cutting-dozens-of-msn-news-production-workers-and-replacing-them-with-artificial-intelligence/.

2. Google Duplex: A.I. Assistant Calls Local Businesses To Make Appointments. (2018). YouTube. Available at: https://www.youtube.com/watch?v=D5VN56jQMWM.

3. Bari Weiss. (n.d.). Resignation Letter. [online] Available at: https://www.bariweiss.com/resignation-letter.

4. Taibbi, M. (2020). The American Press Is Destroying Itself. [online] TK News by Matt Taibbi. Available at: https://taibbi.substack.com/p/the-news-media-is-destroying-itself [Accessed 6 June 2020].

5. Deloitte United States. (2019). Enhancing Digital Fan Engagement. [online] Available at:
    https://www2.deloitte.com/us/en/pages/technology-media-and-telecommunications/articles/enhancing-digital-fan-engagement.html.

6. TOP 5 GLOBAL SPORTS INDUSTRY TRENDS 2. (n.d.). [online] Available at: http://nielsensports.com/wp-content/uploads/2014/09/nielsen-top-5-commercial-sports-trends-2018.pdf.